Dedication

To my gorgeous wife, Tori my love, who has nursed, tended and cared for me, helping me to face the unbearable moments.

❧

ME/Chronic Fatigue Syndrome

A DOCTOR'S JOURNEY

BACK TO HEALTH

'From doctor to patient to doctor again'

STEVEN J. SOMMER M.D.
WITH TORI SOMMER DC

Audiobook and eBook versions available at
drstevensommer.com

A Doctor's Journey Back to Health by Steven J. Sommer M.D.

Copyright 2022 Steven J Sommer, MD. All rights reserved. Except for scholarly fair use and quotations for purposes of review, no part of this book may be reproduced without written permission of the author.

ISBN 978-0-9954345-3-0

Author Portrait by Tori Sommer

DISCLAIMER

This book has been created to bring hope, understanding and direction to individuals (and their families and friends), facing Myalgic Encephalomyelitis/ Chronic Fatigue Syndrome (ME/CFS). It is not intended in any way to replace other professional health care advice, but to support it. Readers of this publication agree that neither Drs Steven and Tori Sommer nor their publisher will be held responsible or liable for damages that may be alleged or resulting, directly, or indirectly, from their use of the information shared in this publication. All external links are provided as a resource only and are not guaranteed to remain active for any length of time. Neither the publisher nor the authors can be held accountable for the information provided by or actions resulting from accessing these resources.

To maintain anonymity, patient's names have been changed.

ALSO, BY DR STEVEN SOMMER

ME/CFS A Path Back to Life - The Art of Micro-Rehab. – Available at www.drstevensommer.com

Finding Hope – Inspiring stories, Healing insights and Health research – book available at www.drstevensommer.com

Restoring Balance – meditation/relaxation-based stress management - CD & MP3 audio recording available at www.drstevensommer.com

ACKNOWLEDGEMENTS

Thank you to all my patients and friends who shared their stories with me so that I could share them with you. I offer particular thanks to Tori Sommer, not just for contributing a chapter to this book, but for her role as a sounding board, editor, narrator and one-person cheer squad when I needed it most. My deepest thanks also to Dr Denise Ruth, Dr Judy Singer, Drs Daniel and Bev Lewis, Dr Vicki Kotsirilos, Dr Joe Di Stefano, Dr Sandra Palmer and Laurie Lacey for their generosity, friendship and help in my hour of need.

To Dr Steven Mitchell, my incredibly skilled dentist who kept my teeth in my mouth through abscesses and root canals, all the while compassionately aware of the bigger picture.

Thank you too to Daniel and Bev Lewis for their friendship, reviewing the manuscript and for contributing a foreword.

The 'Powerful Poets' luncheon lines group meetings where four friends and fellow authors shared our writing, were precious times that kept me on track. Tori, Therese Van Wegen and the late Caspar von Diebitsch; thank you all. A big thank you too to Dr Bambi Ward and the Gador family for their constructive feedback on an earlier draft and Dr David Gallaway and Dr Robin Canniford for proof reading.

My thanks to fellow authors Justine Day, Liz and Alan Flaherty, Liz Manning, Lourdes Llorente, Margot Maurice and her partner John Gallagher, and Christopher Roering for their belief in me as a writer. Margot may no longer be here, but her lessons and spirit of encouragement live on in my heart.

Thanks also to John Garrity for his education, direction and editing and in setting up a home-studio in which Tori could narrate the audiobook.

For the most part, unless published elsewhere, the names and identifying details of the patients and friends mentioned have been changed to preserve anonymity.

CONTENTS

CONTENTS

FOREWORD

DR DANIEL LEWIS RHEUMATOLOGIST

I first met Steven when he was a dynamic medical practitioner and educator championing the benefits of a holistic and integrated approach to health.

He was a lecturer at Monash University, Melbourne and an inspiration to his colleagues and the students he taught. To say that he had a busy life was an understatement.

I lost my connection with him when he became unwell and I heard on the grapevine that he was living in a seaside town in rural Victoria. A year or so later I visited that town and knocked on his front door. I found a man who was a shadow of his former physical self.

Our discussion on that day was possibly the spark of hope that lit the fuse of his subsequent remarkable recovery. A recovery that was not miraculous but the product of his self-research and applying this research in detail and with persistence. The knowledge that Steven has refined is built on his holistic understanding of the human body and mind and his deep connection to mindfulness meditation. This book and the companion book details an approach to recovery that any individual with ME/CFS will relate to and can follow. Further illumination comes from the contribution of Tori, his life partner who cared for him with skill, understanding and unwavering devotion.

From my perspective, the purpose of Steven's work before his illness was to provide better health opportunities for his patients and indirectly to all patients via the doctors and students he taught. Throughout his illness and recovery, his purpose has not wavered.

Steven's vast personal experience and his evidence-based approach to health and healing remain an inspiration to me and to those who know his story.

INTRODUCTION

*"My life with ME/CFS was like living in quicksand.
The more I struggled the more I sank."*

DR STEVEN SOMMER

Myalgic Encephalomyelitis/ Chronic Fatigue Syndrome (ME/CFS), is a World Health Organisation (WHO) classified neurological disorder. Close to two hundred and fifty thousand Australians and millions of people worldwide are afflicted by this disease. Most commonly it is triggered by a virus and is generally considered incurable in all but 5% of people. This said, 40% of people, like myself, do improve; in my case this began after instituting a specific approach to rehabilitation. Before this, ME/CFS had left me unable to work from 1996 to 2004. How I improved enough to be able to return to life and work is the subject of this book.

My story is told alongside the story of ME/CFS, including its history and the fascinating research that's transforming our understanding of this misunderstood illness, research that exposes and **verifies** that ME/CFS is truly a biomedical disease not the psychiatric condition it was once thought to be. It is triggered by a virus in an estimated 80% of people. Viruses implicated include, the Epstein Barr Virus (EBV) which causes mononucleosis, cytomegalovirus (CMV), Ross River Virus and coronaviruses. This is particularly important as indications are SARS-Cov-2, the coronavirus that causes COVID-19, is likely to be such a viral trigger and a percentage of people with Long COVID will go on to become defined as ME/CFS. We'll look at Long COVID in Chapter 7.

A Test?

The research over the last decade is outlined in Chapters 5, 10, 11 and 12. It is likely that this will soon lead to the availability of a simple diagnostic blood test (see Chapter 3). Until this is available the clinical criteria presented in Chapter 3 and Appendix 1 is the gold standard. A diagnostic blood test will be a game changer. Why so? I recently read of a person with Long COVID being told that their troubling symptoms likely result from anxiety, depression, or post-traumatic stress. This is a false and counter-productive attribution that I and countless others with ME/CFS have battled against for years. A test that unequivocally confirms the diagnosis will put to bed this unnecessary and harmful speculation.

An ME/CFS Clinic

When I found a way back to health, I was passionate about helping others who were suffering with this terrible disease and the inappropriate social and medical invalidation that too often accompanies it. So, I ran a dedicated clinic with my wife of 26 years, Tori, for people with ME/CFS. Tori, also my carer throughout my illness, contributes a chapter in the book, *A Carer's Reflection*.

Nothing you can do (?)

This is the message I and many others with ME/CFS have been given. Fortunately, in my previous work as a holistic GP and university lecturer, I had met many people who were told by their doctor(s), regarding other serious illnesses like cancer, 'there's nothing we can do,' yet those people had defied their poor prognoses. I found strength in their courage as they faced their difficulties, embraced life and made positive lifestyle changes.

I soon realized that hope was a very powerful medicine and unless we as humans had hope, whatever life had in store for us would be diminished. Unwittingly some doctors pull the rug of hope out from beneath us. Hence, people were referred to me or 'found' me when they were in dire situations just to have their sense of hope restored.

Through meeting these inspiring people along with my personal experiences, I developed a special interest in mind-body and lifestyle medicine, as I've shared in my book, *Finding Hope*.[1] I effectively became the 'hope' doctor.

What I discovered, though, when I was no longer the doctor, but the patient in the quicksand, was just how difficult it is to see a better future when you're deep in the pit. It was only with Tori's love and the support of special friends and a handful of health practitioners, that I was able to maintain some hope; just. This proved to be a critical foundation for my recovery from ME/CFS.

Origins of this Book

Our clinic closed at the end of 2011 when, due to illnesses and hospitalizations unrelated to ME/CFS, I was once again too sick to work and needed extra care from Tori.[2] Nonetheless, many of my ME/CFS patients were improving with our management strategies. They were some of the most genuine, self-motivated, and yet ill-treated individuals in our society. I felt if I could put what I'd learnt into writing it would allow me to continue to assist them. When the latest recognition that COVID-19 could introduce a whole new subset of those infected with SARS-Cov-2 to long-term ME/CFS, it steeled my determination to get this book (and the next) done, so that I could bring hope and direction from my hard-won lessons learnt both as a doctor and a patient along with Tori's insights.

I began what would be the skeleton of this book in 2012, reviewing my patient files, ME/CFS websites and research journals in the process. More recently I also phoned some of our ex-patients to receive their permission to share their stories and to clarify how they were progressing (most of these stories are shared in my companion book, *ME/CFS – A Path Back to Life*).

Removing Obstacles: A Vital Point About Exercise

For complex reasons, there has been considerable politics surrounding exercise as a management tool in ME/CFS and I devote Chapter 13 to this topic in the hope of removing the obstacles to people with the condition including **appropriate** ME/CFS specific exercise in their management.

The importance and benefit of carefully individualised physical exercise in the management of all neurological disorders is increasingly being recognised. The science of epigenetics may provide a mechanism as to why such a seemingly gentle intervention can assist so much. I devote Chapter 14 to exploring this and the hope it brings to people.

In ME/CFS unlike other neurological diseases, like say Parkinson's disease and MS, an initial period of three to six months of tremendous subtlety in introducing gentle exercise is required to kickstart the body's energy producing mitochondria. If done too quickly cytokine-chemicals will be released into the bloodstream causing post-exertional malaise to last for weeks or months. In this scenario the person with ME/CFS is unlikely to try exercise again! This is a vital point as if done correctly, as outlined in detail in *ME/CFS - A Path Back to life*, enormous benefits are possible, and the person, whilst not cured, can restore much of their life.

Let us begin this exploration with Chris's story, the first person with ME/CFS I'd ever encountered as a GP. The year was 1989, the place, a General Practice clinic in outer suburban Melbourne.

Dr Steven Sommer M.B.,B.S FRACGP
Geelong, March 2022

Chapter 1

ME/CFS CIRCA 1989 - CHRIS'S STORY

"Not being believed," he said,
"was one of the worst experiences of my life."

CHRIS

Before I fell into the debility that was my experience of Chronic Fatigue Syndrome (ME/CFS), I was a practicing General Practitioner (GP) with, I must admit, little knowledge of this condition. All I and indeed many of my colleagues knew was that we did not know if ME/CFS was a 'physical/biomedical' or 'psychological/psychiatric' disease, or simply 'malingering'? There was no definitive specialist or blood test to tell us the answer. Some psychiatrists were telling us it was 'somatisation,' a physical manifestation of a psychiatric problem, others disagreed. Amongst ourselves we would call these unfortunate people our 'heart-sink' patients, because they were clearly suffering and yet we did not know how to help them.

Let me illustrate this with the story of a patient of mine from this time (1989).

Chris's story.

Chris was a 27-year-old man who worked as a security guard for a Bank. His wife Louisa, 25, was a primary school teacher and together they had two young children, Mark, aged 3 and Charlotte 2.

Chris's problems had begun 13 months earlier when he developed a severe sore throat, high fever and extreme fatigue. He saw Dr

I

BD, one of the other five doctors in the GP clinic where I worked, who placed him on the antibiotic Amoxil. Within hours he'd developed a red blotchy skin rash over his entire body. This sort of reaction to Amoxil tends to occur if someone has Infectious Mononucleosis (Glandular Fever), an infection caused by the Epstein Barr virus (EBV). A blood test confirmed that Chris did indeed have this virus, a virus most people catch sometime in their lives, and from which most recover within a few weeks or months. Unfortunately for Chris, over a year later, he was one of the 7% or so who do not fully recover.

I visited his home on a weekend at the end of my Sunday morning clinic session when I was covering for all the other doctors' patients, a six-weekly event. I parked in the driveway of the single-storey, red-brick home. The house may have looked unremarkable from the outside, but that belied the tension mounting within it. I had read Dr BD's notes. Specifically, he had noted that recent blood tests were normal, and they had not shown any re-activation of EBV.

Dr BD had also noted that Chris had not worked for over a year, had applied for, but been rejected by Centrelink for a Disability Support Pension (DSP) and that the family was struggling to keep up their mortgage repayments on Louisa's lone wage. They could no longer afford Child Care, so on weekdays, Louisa had to ask her mother, Maria, who suffered from chronic low back pain, to take care of the kids. Dr BD's final notes about Chris read, '? Malingering.'

I rang the doorbell. Louisa opened it, "Doctor, thank you for coming," she said, her face drawn. "Hello," I said as cheerily as I could muster as she ushered me into the lounge room.

Chris acknowledged me with a faint nod and closed his eyes

again. He was sitting on an armchair, legs elevated. Both kids sat on a rug in front of him and were transfixed by the Wiggles on the screen, the volume unusually low. "Wake up Jeff!" the TV said as loudly as it had been allowed to.

Mark turned to face his dad, "Yeah, wake up Daddy!"

"Yeah," giggled Charlotte. Chris opened his eyes and smiled weakly at the children.

I caught Chris's gaze, but he looked away. Louisa lifted Charlotte on to his knee, then beckoned me into the kitchen.

"He barely moves from there," Louisa said and turned back to face me, "I rang you today, Doctor, as I don't believe Dr BD has any more answers for us. He gave Chris antibiotics, then anti-depressants; it's been a year now, but nothing seems to help." She opened a cupboard and showed me all the bottles of pills. She lowered her voice, "And now Dr BD tells me he agrees with our families that there is nothing wrong with Chris. But why? Look at him, he's sick.... and Chris liked his job, loves me and the kids. He is not doing this because he wants to. What can we do, Doctor?"

"Let me have a look at him," I said and headed back towards Chris in the loungeroom.

"Chris, is there another more private room I can use to examine you?"

"Of course, Doctor," said Chris. Louisa took Charlotte in her arms as Chris rose wearily. He led me to a nearby room and lay down on a bed. I closed the door behind us. I applied a blood pressure cuff and felt his pulse. His heart rate and blood pressure were low. "No fever," I said as I wiped clean the thermometer with an alcohol wipe (the good old days!). Have you always had a slow pulse rate and low blood pressure?" I asked.

3

Chris shrugged his shoulders.

"Do you ever feel dizzy or faint when you stand up?"

He nodded.

I pulled up a chair. "Tell me about what's going on, Chris."

So, he told me his frustrations, told me how useless he felt, how he loved his work, how he hated not being able to support his family.

"Most of all I feel like I'm letting everyone down," Chris said. "My parents don't believe me anymore, neither do Louisa's. Just like Dr BD, they think I'm lazy or 'just depressed.'"

"And what do you think is going on?" I asked.

"I don't know! Isn't that your job, Doc? Why do I sleep 16 hours and wake up tired? Why do I barely have the energy to take a shower? Why, can't I stand loud noises anymore? And every time I try to push myself, I seem to get worse."

I did not know how to answer him. "Have the pills Dr BD gave you helped at all?" was all I could think to ask.

"The anti-depressants?" He looked strangely at me. "Well I'm less depressed but I'm not sure I like it so much..." He lowered his voice, "It's like I'm no better, just as tired and weak, but since I've been taking the pills... I don't... care as much. Is that a good thing Doc?"

"I'll be honest with you, I'm not really sure what's causing this Chris, but I'm going to do some research and I'll call in on you next Friday."

"I'd appreciate that Doc."

"Now can I finish examining you?"

"Sure"

I found nothing else of significance and left Chris resting. I met
Louisa in the kitchen, Mark and Charlotte in front of the kitchen
bench on the lounge room floor, still watching TV.

"What are we going to do?" Louisa pleaded.

"Look," I said. "I'm not sure what's going on but like you, I believe
Chris. After all what has he to gain by staying sick. I've told
him I will do some research and call in on Friday at the end of
my session."

"Thank you, Doctor."

I left knowing that whatever was ailing Chris was destroying not
only him but his family too. I was determined to find out what it was
and how I could help him overcome it.

As things turned out, Louisa called the next day to tell me that
a friend of hers travelling through the UK had related Chris's
story to a nurse she knew, who suggested it might be Myalgic
Encephalomyelitis (ME), the term used in the UK for ME/CFS. She
suggested they find a support group.

"What do you think Doctor?"

"I'll look into it, Louisa and call you back this evening." I had a
busy schedule that day, so I asked the ever-reliable Joanne, the
practice nurse, whether she could do some homework for me. By
day's end she'd found a reputable ME/CFS support group and I
passed this information on to Chris and Louisa that night.

When I saw the family again that Friday the squeezing tension
there just five days ago had eased, hope had re-entered the
household. A man called Jim had spoken with them over the
phone, reassuring them that Chris was not alone with this sort of
problem. He invited them to attend the local support group.

Never could I have imagined back then just how terrible this lack of validation would feel, or that a support group could be so important. Soon I would be the one on the other side of the desk seeking similar validation and answers. When I became one of these unfortunate people the treatment I received, not just from colleagues, but family and friends, was frankly, with few exceptions, shocking. It has left scars. I decided then and there that if I ever became well enough to return to work, I would set up a clinic to care for people who had fallen through the medical cracks with ME/CFS. It gave me a reason to fight.

Chapter 2

A BRIEF HISTORY OF ME/CFS

"Those who do not learn (from) history are doomed to repeat it."

GEORGE SANTAYANA - PHILOSOPHER

In 1800 BC a Babylonian philosopher king, known as Hammurabi, described an illness involving chronic full bodily intolerance of exercise, a hallmark of ME/CFS.[1] In more modern times Charles Darwin, who recorded his personal health experiences in his journals, describes a chronic 'wretched' illness with ME/CFS like qualities.[2]

In 1869 a diagnosis of neurasthenia was popularized by American psychiatrist George Beard. The condition described by Beard also had some similarities to ME/CFS.

It is also possible that the heroic British nurse Florence Nightingale became ill with neurasthenia (ME/CFS) after returning from her work during the Crimean War (1853-56). After her time in Crimea, she was mythologised as 'the Lady with the Lamp' as she'd carried a lamp through the darkness on her nightly ward rounds bringing comfort and assistance to the injured soldiers. After the war she spent years housebound and often bedbound. Too exhausted to speak to more than one person at a time, she'd receive visits from politicians at her bedside. Despite these limitations she continued to write, lobbying for better healthcare for soldiers and civilians alike.

Florence Nightingale's risk profile for developing neurasthenia would be quite typical for someone with ME/CFS today. Exposure to many infectious diseases, notably Q Fever,[3] exhausting physical work and little time for rest in emotionally stressful circumstances.

Epidemics

Although ME/CFS most commonly occurs sporadically, that is, in isolated cases like MS or Parkinson's Disease, unlike these diseases, it can also occur in epidemics. An epidemic suggests a highly infectious trigger. The history of recorded outbreaks of epidemic ME/CFS has been documented more than 60 times since 1934. Most of the classic descriptions of ME/CFS have come from people affected in these epidemics. The four examples listed in Table 1 came from a time before Jonas Salk's poliomyelitis (Polio) vaccine became available in the mid to late 1950's, so some of these epidemics were originally thought to be Polio.[4]

Los Angeles County General Hospital in 1934
Iceland 1948/9
Adelaide (Australia) 1949-1951
London's Royal Free Hospital in 1955
Table 1 Four of over 60 Documented ME/CFS Epidemics since 1934.

Polio is a potentially life-threatening illness caused by an enterovirus, that is, a virus transmitted through our gut wall via faecal (poo) contaminated water or food and potentially causing paralysis. With the discovery of a virus that could affect the nervous system, as in people with Polio, it was thought for a while that ME/CFS might have a similar, singular viral cause.[5] However, in ME/CFS no common infectious agent has been found, with multiple viruses including some similar enteroviruses (polio-like), Epstein Barr Virus (EBV – which causes Infectious Mononucleosis/ Glandular Fever) and Cytomegalovirus (CMV) being implicated.

Of great interest is the Polio epidemic that occurred in Iceland in 1955, seven years after a documented ME/CFS epidemic in 1948 had swept through various districts on the island. No one on the island had yet received the Salk polio vaccine and yet people living in those districts who had been exposed to the ME/CFS epidemic seven years earlier did not contract polio. This implies that whichever virus was responsible for the earlier ME/CFS epidemic in 1948 had been similar enough to provide immunity, a natural vaccination if you like, against the enterovirus that caused Polio in 1955.[6]

There are other possible connections between ME/CFS and Polio. Before the Salk vaccine, the responses to the polio virus in different people exposed to this infection ranged from paralysis and death to a milder version known as Non-Paralytic Polio (NPP). Up to 40 years after an NPP infection, some people who had experienced this milder form of Polio went on to develop an illness with similarities to ME/CFS known as Post-Polio Syndrome (PPS). Like ME/CFS the precise mechanism that causes PPS is unknown. Yet it shares many features with ME/CFS, the key difference being it tends to be progressive and as in the original disease can cause permanent loss of muscle strength that, unlike ME/CFS, does not restore with carefully administered exercise.[7]

What about Coronavirus?

The deadly 'SARS' (coronavirus SARS-CoV-1) epidemic of 2003 (see Chapter 7) killed around 10% of the 8000 people who were infected. It also left around 20 to 30% of those who recovered unable to return to full time work one to two years later due to symptoms consistent with ME/CFS. Whilst the current SARS-CoV-2 is less deadly per infection at an estimated 1 to 4% mortality rate, it has proven to be far more infectious infecting millions across the globe causing the first global pandemic in a century. New strains have become even more infectious and some more deadly.

As we will explore in Chapter 7, there is already evidence of chronic health problems in COVID-19 survivors, these complications following the resolution of the acute illness include an ME/CFS-like disease.

Sadly, there are already reports of some people with this post viral (long-Covid) syndrome being told that their troubling ongoing symptoms are likely to result from anxiety, depression, or post-traumatic stress.[8] Bizarrely, this ongoing 'psychologising' of post-viral syndromes like ME/CFS continues despite the fact that research, as you'll see in upcoming chapters, does not support this psychological diagnosis. In fact, as I've said, it has been classified as a neurological disease by the WHO and its International Classification of Diseases (ICD-8 G93.3) since 1969.

Why this continuing craziness I hear you ask? Well, it appears to have its origins in the United Kingdom.

The Hysteria Myth

The most well-known and studied example of epidemic ME/CFS in the UK occurred in 1955. Nearly 300 members of the hospital staff at London's Royal Free Hospital developed what was obviously an infectious illness with fever over a period of four and half months. Of the ill hospital staff, 255 were so ill they had to be admitted to the hospital as patients. Typical of ME/CFS, many of these staff remained unwell for the rest of their lives.[9]

In 1970, two British psychiatrists, Colin McEvedy and William Beard, following what most now would consider grossly inadequate research, had two papers published in the British Medical Journal: 'Royal Free Epidemic of 1955: a reconsideration,' and 'Concept of Benign Myalgic Encephalomyelitis.'[10]

In these articles they proposed that the Royal Free Hospital Epidemic of 1955 had been an outbreak of mass hysteria, and that other outbreaks in the world also had features of hysteria. When they wrote these articles, neither of them had bothered to interview or examine any of the Royal Free staff who had been involved, some of whom were still unwell 15 years later (i.e. in 1970).

There were obvious flaws in their methodology and reasoning. Documented signs of infection, such as fever, and neurological involvement do not occur in hysteria. Yet this psychiatric hypothesis was taken up by the media. Unfortunately, it was also accepted without question by many of the medical profession, even to this day! The trivialization and inappropriate management of ME/CFS that has resulted from this, has done and continues to do incalculable damage.[11]

As Chapters 10 through 12 will attest the scientific evidence is well and truly in and it's time to cremate this outdated and preposterous hysteria hypothesis.

❦

Let me complete this history lesson with a summary of how doctors have viewed ME/CFS over the ages:

- 1800 BC - first noted by Hammurabi in Babylon. He observed and recorded a description of, what we'd call in modern-day terms, a 'chronic systemic exertional intolerance' disease.
- Late 19th century – labelled by the name 'Neurasthenia', an illness Charles Darwin and Florence Nightingale may have had.
- 1930 – CFS thought to be a form of Polio – named Myalgic Encephalomyelitis (ME) in 1955 after the Royal Free Hospital Epidemic.
- 1969 - The World Health Organization's International Classification of Diseases (ICD-8) classifies ME/CFS as a neurological illness (G93.3).

- 1984 – named Chronic Fatigue Syndrome (CFS).
- 1970 to 2014 – A poorly researched hypothesis by two psychiatrists published in 1970, suggested ME/CFS was in fact the psychiatric condition of 'Hysteria.' This suggestion spread hysterically and persists to this day. Eventually it morphed into a more sophisticated cognitive-behavioural model, which attributes the symptoms and debility purely as the result of deconditioning, originating from patients' fear of activity and false cognitions.
- 2003 SARS-CoV-1 leaves around 25% of survivors unable to return to full time work due to an ME/CFS-like illness one to two years later.
- 2015 – ME/CFS confirmed as biomedical (neuroimmune), not psychiatric, after 23 studies consistently demonstrate post exertional malaise correlates with abnormal immune responses, including cytokine patterns/algorithms. The independent non-profit Institute of Medicine in the USA (now called National Academy of Medicine) proposes renaming ME/CFS as Systemic Exertional Intolerance Disease (SEID), as Hammurabi had noted 3,800 years ago! (This is explored in more detail in Chapter 12).
- 2010 to 2021 – More sophisticated research tools have provided significant evidence of neurological, immunological, autonomic and energy metabolism impairment in people with ME/CFS. In Chapters 5, 10-12, we will explore this in some depth.
- 2018 - The World Health Organization's International Classification of Diseases (ICD-11) continues to classify ME/CFS as a neurological illness (G93.3).

- 2019 – SARS-CoV-2 pandemic is leaving many with long-COVID syndrome, a post-viral illness that in a proportion of people, after six months, is fitting the criteria of ME/CFS (see Chapter 3 & Appendix 1) and affecting millions of people world-wide.

Chapter 2
Key Points

✓ Babylonian records suggest ME/CFS may have occurred 3,800 years ago.

✓ Neurasthenia was a name given to a condition that may have been ME/CFS like in the late 19th century.

✓ Charles Darwin may have suffered from this 'wretched' illness.

✓ Florence Nightingale remained house and often bedbound for the last 10 years of her life with neurasthenia.

✓ ME/CFS usually occurs in individuals sporadically, like other neurological conditions (e.g. Multiple Sclerosis and Parkinson's Disease). However, there have also been over 60 recorded epidemics of ME/CFS since 1934. An epidemic strongly suggests an infectious cause.

✓ Viruses implicated as triggering the onset of ME/CFS include EBV, CMV, enteroviruses and coronaviruses, including the original SARS virus, SARS-CoV-1, and it appears, the virus that causes COVID-19, SARS-CoV-2.

✓ Although the exact effect may take years to calculate, it appears likely that the current pandemic will leave behind many people unwell with post COVID 19 illnesses that include ME/CFS, with a significant number unable to work.

✓ Supporting the hypothesis that a virus like the Polio enterovirus was one potential cause of ME/CFS, is the documentation in Iceland of an epidemic of an ME/CFS-like illness in 1948. In the districts in which this occurred no one contracted Polio when an outbreak of Polio swept through the island in 1955. (Note: There was no polio vaccine available at the time.) The implication being that in 1948 a similar virus to the Polio enterovirus was involved and had transmitted immunity, much like the Salk Polio Vaccine would do a decade later, against contracting polio.

✓ In 1970 two British psychiatrists McEvedy and Beard published a hypothesis implying epidemics of ME/CFS were due to hysteria. There was no research to support this, yet the idea took hold amongst the general and medical populations alike. The trivialization and inappropriate management of ME/CFS that has resulted from this has done and continues to do incalculable damage.

✓ The World Health Organisation (WHO) International Classification of Diseases (ICD) continues to classify ME/CFS as a neurological disease.

Chapter 3

DIAGNOSIS, PREVALENCE AND PROGNOSIS

"To not have your suffering recognized is an almost unbearable form of violence."

ANDREI LANKOV
NORTH KOREAN EXPERT KOOKMIN UNIVERSITY SOUTH KOREA.

Apart from the names Chronic Fatigue Syndrome (CFS) and Myalgic Encephalomyelitis (ME), in the USA ME/CFS has also been known as Chronic Fatigue Immune Deficiency Syndrome (CFIDS) and more recently as Systemic Exertion Intolerance Disease (SEID). It is classified by the World Health Organization as a disease of the central nervous system[1] characterized by debilitating fatigue that is not relieved with rest and is associated with a range of other physical symptoms that we will explore below.

Diagnosis

There is no simple diagnostic test yet for ME/CFS (although more complex testing does reveal consistent abnormalities – more on this in Chapters 10-12), so for now, at least, the diagnosis is based on symptoms. This is not unusual for neurological diseases. For example, there is currently no definitive test for Parkinson's disease.

In terms of ME/CFS, several different symptom-based criteria models have been proposed over the years in order to pin down a diagnosis. These include the Fukuda and International Clinical Criteria. Some still argue that ME and CFS are different illnesses,[2] although most now accept them as one in the same.

I will use the term ME/CFS as defined by the 2003 Canadian Diagnostic Clinical Criteria (CDCC) - See Appendix 1. This is the diagnostic criteria I used in my clinic and one that most current researchers into ME/CFS use, although in 2015 the National Academy of Medicine (NAM) in the US came up with a more succinct approach than the CDCC. These NAM criteria are becoming more widely accepted. While the name change of Systemic Exertional Intolerance Disease (SEID) was also proposed at this time, it was not adopted, so that ME/CFS remains the accepted name.

A consensus review of ME/CFS by 21 physicians published on August 2021 by the Mayo Clinic advises physicians to use the NAM criteria outlined in Table 1.[3]

ME/CFS

The **diagnosis** requires that the unwell person have the following 3 symptoms:

1. FATIGUE – A substantial reduction or impairment in the ability to engage in pre-illness levels of occupational, educational, social, or personal activities, that persists for more than 6 months (3 months in children). The fatigue is often profound of new or definite onset (not lifelong), is not the result of ongoing excessive exertion, and is not substantially alleviated by rest.
2. Post Exertional Malaise (PEM)
3. Unrefreshing Sleep

One of the two following manifestations is also required:

1. Cognitive Impairment
2. Orthostatic Intolerance

NOTE: The diagnosis of ME/CFS should be questioned if people **do not** have these symptoms with moderate, substantial, or severe intensity for at least half of the time.

Table 1 ME/CFS Diagnostic Criteria
(National Academy of Sciences/Medicine 2015)[4]

To contrast, the Canadian Diagnostic Clinical Criteria that I used in my clinic for five years is presented in Appendix 1. I include a look at it as it gives you a broader sense of the variety of symptoms people with ME/CFS can experience. This breadth of symptoms reflects a multisystem disease that is often physically, mentally and emotionally debilitating. The fact that people with this diagnosis are twice as likely to be unemployed as people with fatigue who do not meet these formal criteria for ME/CFS,[5] is demonstrative of its seriousness, the implications of which we will explore shortly.

There are some conditions that can mimic ME/CFS, hence a definitive diagnosis can only be confirmed when these other disease processes are excluded; clinical examination, blood tests, and if indicated, other specialized tests for causes of severe fatigue, like sleep apnea, being negative.[6] (See Appendix 2).

Central Sensitivity Syndromes

It is also important to note that ME/CFS can co-exist with a variety of comorbidities including the Central Sensitivity Syndromes that relate to chronic pain, such as, fibromyalgia, chronic headaches, irritable bowel syndrome, temporomandibular disorder (see Appendix 4). In these Central Sensitivity Syndromes the brain is inappropriately signaling in response to various inputs.[7] Functional brain imaging has confirmed over-responsive areas in people with these syndromes,[8] effectively indicating a neurological malfunction.

Out of these Central Sensitivity Syndromes, fibromyalgia, is commonly mistaken for ME/CFS. Although the two can co-exist, fibromyalgia's main distinguishing feature is a predominance of muscle pain over fatigue. There is also more likelihood of PEM, brain fog, low blood pressure and immune system problems in ME/CFS than in people with fibromyalgia.[9-11]

We will explore brain imaging findings in ME/CFS in Chapter 5.

Post Exertional Malaise (PEM)

Of all the symptoms presented in Table 1, the most cardinal symptom of ME/CFS is post-exertional malaise (PEM). This is characterized by extreme fatigue, pain, cognitive deficits and other symptoms flaring after a level of exertion (physical or mental/emotional) that would previously have been easily tolerated.

PEM and Energy Metabolism Impairment

In most healthy and sick people, physical exercise improves fatigue, sleep, pain, cognition, and mood.[12-15] By contrast, people with ME/CFS with PEM experience a distinctive exacerbation of symptoms and a further reduction in functioning after previously tolerated exertion. Multiple studies using both patient-reported and physiologic outcome measures have confirmed this.[16-19]

While post-exercise fatigue and musculoskeletal pain are common in healthy people and other medical conditions (e.g. osteoarthritis), **the post-exertional worsening of function** and the **constellation of symptoms** (such as sleep, memory, concentration, flu-like feelings [eg, sore throat], and mood) seen in ME/CFS **are distinctive**.

Most commonly PEM symptoms tend to be identical to those of the original triggering illness minus any fever if there ever was one. PEM is also characterized by an unusually slow recovery to baseline, not explained by deconditioning, sedentary lifestyle or malingering.[20] This return to baseline can take hours, days, weeks or even months. Another important aspect of PEM is that the **onset can often be delayed and begin 24-48 hours post-exertion**. This onset delay might help establish a differential diagnosis between ME/CFS and other diseases, such as, Multiple Sclerosis and Lupus, that can have severe fatigue and malaise after overexertion but no delay of onset.[21]

Up until the three-month (children) or six-month (adults) duration, the illness may often be labelled as 'post-viral fatigue'. In societies which rarely allow more than two weeks off work or study due to sickness, it is thought that at least some people who have post-viral fatigue could prevent their ill-health worsening or developing further into ME/CFS if they could somehow find a way to rest adequately and not push themselves too hard physically or mentally early on. This would allow their body to rest and recover adequately from what could otherwise become the initiating illness.

On the other hand, there are some people with ME/CFS who become so fearful of PEM, that they can become wary of any movement or exertion aggravating their situation through lack of activity. We will look at how both these unhelpful responses i.e. pushing through fatigue while ill or too little activity, can be better managed in the companion book *ME/CFS – A Path Back to Life - The Art of Micro-Rehab*.

Orthostatic Intolerance

Orthostatic intolerance (OI) refers to a fall in blood pressure when standing or in some people just sitting upright. It can be very debilitating and can cause one to feel dizzy, fatigued, light-headed, palpitations, sore legs or faint and reduce cognitive ability.[22] See: https://www.dysautonomiainternational.org/pdf/RoweOIsummary.pdf

It occurs in 95% of people with ME/CFS and is caused by a malfunctioning autonomic nervous system.[23] This malfunction is thought to be triggered by a virus and/or an abnormal immune response. A current example is infection with the coronavirus, SARS Cov 2. Research is showing that those who go onto develop long-COVID (around 10% of those infected) also show signs of orthostatic intolerance that they didn't have prior to being infected.[24] Of these people, those who continue to have symptoms beyond six months will no longer be defined as long-COVID but as ME/CFS.[25] We will look at this in more detail in Chapters 6 and 7.

My personal experience with OI was that I struggled to stand still for more than a few minutes due to sore calves and dizziness. This was quickly relieved by sitting or lying down with my legs elevated on a cushion. Some people with ME/CFS also experience subtler symptoms, such as feeling sick, nauseous, tired, or confused during periods of sitting upright or standing still. It is sometimes misinterpreted as anxiety, but this can easily be sorted out with specific blood pressure testing as outlined below.

The 10 Minute NASA Lean Test

The 10-minute NASA Lean Test is currently the recommended version of a standing blood pressure test. It was developed by The Bateman Horne Clinic in the USA (see www.BatemanHorneCenter.org). It has been used to assess the presence and/or severity of orthostatic intolerance in thousands of people since the year 2000. This is what to expect (See Table 2:

- You will be asked to remove your shoes, socks and any pressure stockings you may have on. You may also be asked to cease certain fluids and medications [Note: Do not do this unless instructed to by your prescribing doctor.]
- Under medical supervision you will then be asked to lie down flat on your back on an examination couch (i.e. in a supine-face upward position).
- Your blood pressure and heart rate will be recorded every minute.
- Once two very similar readings are attained, you will be asked to stand up straight, feet flat on the floor, leaning your back against a wall for support.

Once again, your blood pressure and heart rate will be recorded every minute, for a further 10 minutes. If you feel unwell before this ten-minutes ends, let the supervising practitioner know.

Table 2. Instructions for NASA Lean Test

Another test that can be used to confirm the presence or otherwise of orthostatic intolerance is a Tilt Table Test. This is usually performed in specialist cardiology labs.

A Simple Blood Test?

A much easier way to diagnose the condition may not be far away. Researchers at Griffith University in Australia have discovered a defective calcium ion receptor on the surface of immune cells in people with ME/CFS. This impairs the movement of calcium from outside the cell to inside the cell which is likely to have global ill-effects throughout the body.[26] They are confident that this discovery will translate within a few years to a simple blood test that would be able to diagnose ME/CFS.[27]

As we'll see in chapters 10-12, the race is on for the first research team to develop a diagnostic blood test.

How Common is ME/CFS?

ME/CFS occurs in two peak age groups, 10 to 19 years and 30 to 39 years with an average age of 33.[28] It can occur in people as young as 2 years or as old as 77 years. It is three times as likely to occur in women than men, although there is no gender difference in incidence when it occurs in children. It is estimated more than 2.5 million Americans and over 250,000 Australians are living with ME/CFS.[29,30,31] However, it is conceivable in countries who've taken a big hit from COVID-19, like the UK and USA, that these numbers could more than double despite increasing vaccination rates, as the conversion from acute to chronic disease is already in train in millions already COVID infected.

Before the COVID-19 pandemic ME/CFS tended to occur sporadically. In other words, it was not contagious of itself, much as say Parkinson's disease isn't, but as we explored in Chapter 2, it has occurred in epidemics (clusters) in the past following outbreaks of particularly nasty viral infections. Hence, this current pandemic SARS-Cov-2 virus could result in a huge increase in the number of people being left behind with ME/CFS or an ME/CFS-like illness. We'll explore this further in Chapter 7.

Social and Economic Impact

Unlike the false past-perception of it being "yuppy flu" and only affecting the worried and wealthy well, ME/CFS favors neither social class, race nor culture.[32-37] Fame doesn't make you immune to it either. For example, it has affected international entertainers Cher, Sinead O'Connor and Michael Crawford. Other well-known people include Laura Hillenbrand – author of *Seabiscuit*, Pema Chodron author and Buddhist nun and numerous professional athletes (we look at the story of Australian Rules footballer Alastair Lynch in *ME/CFS – A Path Back to Life – The Art of Micro-Rehab*).

As a severely debilitating chronic disease, ME/CFS places a tremendous burden on people affected by it and their caregivers, as well as the health care system. Unemployment rates among those with the disorder range from 35% to 69%. One US study found individual income losses of approximately $20,000 annually occurred in households[38,39] affected by ME/CFS.

The Canadian Community Health Survey of 2005 and 2010 documented people affected by ME/CFS were significantly more impaired compared to many Canadians with other chronic conditions, such as cancer and heart disease. Those with ME/CFS reported high levels of permanent inability to work, needing help with activities of daily living and a high number of consultations with doctors (10+ per year). They reported high rates (29%) of unmet health care and home care needs and high levels (20%) of moderate or severe food insecurity, indicating they were unable to access sufficiently affordable or nutritious food. Reasons beyond affordability included not having the energy to go shopping or prepare home cooked meals, let alone washing up!

Other Canadian studies confirm an income and productivity loss of $20,000 per person with ME/CFS, and many report an annual household income less than $15,000, as many, like Tori did for me, had to reduce or quit work in order to care for their loved one.[40-42] In the US between 836,000 to 2.5 million people have ME/CFS, with the direct and indirect economic costs to society estimated to be in the billions; somewhere between $18 and $24 billion annually.[43]

Prognosis

Patients most commonly report a fluctuating illness pattern in which symptoms wax and wane but are always present. The long-term prognosis of ME/CFS is variable, with children having a better recovery rate than adults. Most adults affected by ME/CFS show some improvement over the first five years of the illness but usually plateau out below their pre-illness functioning level. Most of these people never regain their previous level of health or functioning.[44,45]

In terms of the stats, although it is known that patients can be ill for years or even decades, no definitive study of prognosis exists. Studies are limited by small sample sizes, high dropout rates, short follow-up times, inclusion of patients with other conditions, and inappropriate definitions of recovery.[46]

This said, the statistics we do have for adults affected by ME/CFS are sobering. A review of 14 studies found on average that **just 5%** of patients considered themselves completely recovered (range 0%–31%); 40% of patients improved during follow-up (range 8%–63%); only

8%–30% who lost the ability to work were able to return to work; and 5%–20% of patients reported ongoing worsening of symptoms.[47-49]

Cox and Findley summarise the wide range of key limitations a person with ME/CFS can face or cycle back and forth through in Table 3.[50]

- **Mild**: mobile and self-caring; may continue working but will have reduced other activities due to the need to rest more.
- **Moderate**: reduced mobility, restricted in basic activities of daily living, such as showering, dressing, meal prep etc needs frequent periods of rest; usually not working.
- **Severe**: mostly housebound; limited to minimal activities of daily living (eg, face washing, showering); severe cognitive difficulties; may be wheelchair dependent.
- **Very severe**: mostly bedridden; unable to independently carry out most activities of daily living; often experience extreme sensitivity to light, sound, and other sensory input.
- **Overall:** up to 75% are unable to work, and an estimated 25% are consistently housebound or bedbound.[51,52] The level of severity can fluctuate, with 61% reporting being bedbound on their worst days.[53]

Table 3 Classification by Severity

In practical terms at any one time, like Chris whose story we explored in Chapter 1, about a quarter of people affected by ME/CFS will be largely housebound or bedbound due to the disease's severity. About 25% will have a milder condition allowing them to at least participate in part-time work or school, whilst around 50% will be somewhere between these two ranges of functioning.[54,55] Many remain unwell and have frequent relapses for the rest of their lives. During the course of the illness, people affected by ME/CFS commonly have good (remission) and bad (relapse) days, a boom and bust cycle, with bad days being called 'crash' days.[56] Even those who do largely recover often still need more rest than their contemporaries.

It is worth noting that on bad days, the degree of impairment can exceed that of rheumatoid arthritis, multiple sclerosis, depression, heart disease, cancer, and lung disease.[57-59]

Now it is recognized as a life-long neuroimmune condition which can wax and wane, like MS, this helps to explain the behavior of this disease. We are beginning to uncover how this is occurring in the body and with greater understanding will come better treatments. In *ME/CFS A Path Back to Life - The Art of Micro-Rehab*, we'll explore ways that can improve your life right now.

Factors known to increase the risk of ending up with a more severe level of illness are:[60-62]

- The severity of the initiating illness.
- Severe orthostatic intolerance, for example, feeling faint with a high risk of falling due to low blood pressure on standing.
- The standard of early management of the illness (e.g. late diagnosis or frequent overexertion in the early stages of the illness are likely to lead to deterioration).
- Having a family history, especially a mother with the illness.
- A diagnosis of fibromyalgia together with ME/CFS.

Chapter 3
Key Points

✓ ME/CFS also goes by the names Myalgic Encephalomyelitis (ME), Chronic Fatigue Syndrome (ME/CFS), Chronic Fatigue Immune Deficiency Syndrome (CFIDS) and Systemic Exertion Intolerance Disease (SEID). It is classified by the World Health Organization as a disease of the central nervous system.

✓ There is no simple diagnostic test, although there are promising possibilities (see Chapter 12). Currently, the diagnosis of ME/CFS is guided by the exclusion of other possible causes of these symptoms (via adequate assessment that will include physical examination and medical tests) and the inclusion of the symptoms outlined in the NAM criteria (see Table 1 and Appendices 1 and 2). The 10-minute NASA Lean Test performed in a medical clinic can help to diagnose the illness and determine its severity by detection of orthostatic intolerance, present in 95% of people with ME/CFS.

✓ Apart from looking closely at the NAM Diagnostic criteria in Table 1, if you haven't already, it is worth taking a close look at Appendix 1 (Canadian Diagnostic Criteria) to clarify the large range of body systems that can be affected.

✓ Delayed onset post exertional malaise (PEM) is defining of this illness. The symptoms during a PEM relapse tend to be identical to the original illness but without any fever.

✓ The social and economic impact of this disease can be devastating, sending families, (like Chris's – see Chapter 1; and Tori and I – Chapters 4, 8, 9 into unemployment and poverty.

✓ The severity prevalence is such that at any one time 25% will be housebound or bedbound, 25% will have a milder version allowing them to at least hold down a part-time job or study, while the other 50% will be somewhere in between.

Chapter 4

MY TIPPING POINT

"Midway this way of life we're bound upon,
I woke to find myself in a dark wood,
where the right road was wholly lost and gone."

DANTE THE DIVINE COMEDY – HELL

Let me share my ME/CFS story with you, beginning with the last time I felt fully fit and strong. It was July 1992, I was 31-years old and my career as a medical educator was taking off…

The hum of the aircraft comforted me as I sat back contemplating the weekend ahead. The five-hour flight from Melbourne to Darwin gave me plenty of time to reflect on my strategy. It was a big moment for me. In my fourth year at Monash University's Department of Community Medicine (General Practice), I had recently passed my Fellowship of the Royal Australian College of General Practitioners (FRACGP) examinations and been promoted to a senior lecturer position. This trip to Darwin was the most responsibility I had been given yet. A dozen foreign medical graduates were waiting for me to conduct a full weekend of training to prepare them for the tough examinations they would need to pass if they were to practice medicine in Australia. The Federal Government was paying our department to do this, and I was given the job.

Carousels of slides and multiple handouts filled my suitcase, still years before the wondrous PowerPoint, USB sticks and The Cloud. I would be conducting tutorials and ward rounds in Darwin hospital, teaching not only clinical skills but exam technique, critical to their chances of success in a foreign country. It was an intense trial for them. For some this would be their last chance to practice medicine. For me, improving their communication and clinical skills whilst acclimatizing them to Australian expectations and exams was a challenge I relished.

Disembarking from the plane onto the tarmac, I breathed in the warmth of the tropics. There's something especially relaxing about that first breath of warm air when you've been living and breathing in a cold winter. It'd been 8°C (46°F) when the plane left Melbourne and arriving to a 24°C (75°F) balmy evening was a definite perk from this job.

After checking in at the hotel, there was little time to rest; a Friday night dinner had been arranged with overseas and local doctors in my honour and was to be followed by my first lecture. I loved teaching, it was the reason I went for the job at the University and I ripped into it with gusto; demonstrating techniques, emphasising culturally sensitive bedside manner, answering questions and finishing sessions with mini-exams to consolidate their learning.

The weekend was long and demanding but I was energized and gratified from teaching such an eager to learn group of doctors. Most exciting of all, my then girlfriend and future wife to be, Tori, joined me in Darwin on the Sunday evening. Neither of us had holidayed here before and we looked forward to exploring this beautiful part of the world.

The next day we hired a campervan and began our travels through Kakadu National Park. A glorious holiday whose colours remain etched in our memories. Perfect weather, camping by and swimming in water holes (picture Crocodile Dundee); there are not enough words to describe its many delights. It proved to be an experience of a lifetime.

✀

By the end of that year (1992) my energy was beginning to falter. I'd developed pneumonia in October and this was complicated with my first asthma episodes. Some fatigue persisted until the end of November, so I decided to halve my workload at the University and focus more on my General Practice work.

It's worth pointing out my workload at this time consisted of a full-time university position that incorporated general practice work, four sessions a week. I had also begun to run stress management groups and presentations both at the clinic, Uni and elsewhere and was a board member of the non-profit educational organization, the Whole Health Institute of Australasia (WHI). Focusing on the common ground of caring and a holistic approach to healing, WHI broke down the barriers between people and particularly between various mainstream and complementary health professionals. In the 1990's it was counter-culture to the business model that was growing in Medicine, and I felt a little like a revolutionary.

My reduced workload didn't last long. By early 1993 WHI's president had retired and I had been asked to step in to fill the breach, which I did. My stress management consultancy work was also growing, and I began to give presentations throughout Australia. I was internally driven to make a difference to help people and I loved doing so.

Tori and I got engaged and moved in together. I attempted to balance my output by practicing an hour and a half of yoga and meditation each morning at 6.00 AM. Tori and I also swam 1 km three times per week at a local pool and walked to the beach from our apartment most evenings. Despite these measures, my health continued to gradually decline as I seemed to 'collect' more illnesses each year.

At the end of 1993 I was invited to present a paper at the second Dead Sea Scrolls conference in Tiberius, by the Sea of Galilee in Israel. The paper outlined the ground-breaking work Dr Craig Hassed and I were doing with medical students, introducing them to a mindfulness meditation-based stress management program. Craig could not go so

I said yes. Tori pleaded with me not to attend the conference as she could see I was exhausted and needed my holiday-time to rest and recharge. Keen to present my paper and to catch up with my Israeli relatives, I ignored her sage advice; if only I'd known how much payback was coming!

Within hours of arrival in Israel I experienced back spasms followed by a nasty upper respiratory infection and asthma. I struggled on, managed to present my paper and after the conference, took a bus from Tiberius to Jerusalem to visit family and friends. I hadn't had time to stop and was feeling very hungry, so against my better instincts I purchased a falafel with a rich tahini sauce from a street-side vendor (the Israeli equivalent to a veggie burger). That night I experienced a bout of severe food poisoning, which would turn out to be the beginning trigger for an unrequited relationship with Irritable Bowel Syndrome (IBS).

When I returned home, it was apparent to me and Tori that I'd lost another level of physical health. I was tiring more easily and sleeping more. I saw my GP again and had various tests that came back 'normal.' Still, I enjoyed my work with its variety and carried on with gusto and albeit a few more visits to the loo!

❦

Tori and I were married on a hot summer's day in December 1994. The garden wedding took place at her grandparent's bluestone home in Batesford, just outside of Geelong, Victoria. It was a beautiful, memorable day. We married under a Peppercorn tree, with violins playing. Our marriage celebrant, Lance, confirmed our union, timber resonating from his Canadian accented voice.

It was a hot day, barely a breath of wind with temperatures reaching 33 C (91 F). Neither of us is religious but for me and my family's sake we added a few Jewish components like breaking the glass and a circle

Hora dance with lots of 'spinning around' that in the heat turned into a 'horror' dance leaving me wretching and nauseated.

Fortunately, one of the guests, a fellow GP, had his Doctor's Bag with him and an IV dose of Maxolon allowed me to recover enough to give my speech.

Our wedding night at a nearby Bed & Breakfast in the countryside was memorable for all the wrong reasons. At 1.00am I woke with a severe asthma attack. Tori had to drive me into the ER at the Hospital to be treated.

Our honeymoon driving tour of New Zealand that immediately followed, was notable for how much time I needed to rest. A swim with the dolphins at Kaikoura near the top of the South-island turned into a nightmare as I became severely seasick and then hypothermic almost requiring hospitalization. I had to be wrapped in multiple blankets and a doona with the heaters up to max once we got back to our hotel room. Even with hot drinks it took three exhausting hours for me to stop shivering. We slowed down our activities after that and by the end of our five-week sojourn I was better but clearly not back to health.

Still, unconscious of what would soon befall me, I barreled into 1995 'saving the world,' all the while continuing to lose stamina. By year's end I could only swim half of the 1 km distance I'd previously swum continuously and even this, only by stopping to rest after each lap. My general practitioner (GP) had ordered new blood tests but nothing obvious was found to explain my ongoing decline. A gluten and lactose-free diet and detoxification program did improve my IBS but by the time 1996 came around, I needed to rest all weekend just to make it back to work each Monday morning.

A Mediation Role

In the middle of that fateful year (1996), I was asked to chair a mediation between two groups of doctors competing with each other; The Australian Complementary Medicine Association (ACMA), headed by Dr Mark Donohue, and the Australian Integrative Medicine Association (AIMA), led by Dr Vicki Kotsirilos. The Federal Government wanted to deal with a single body to represent doctors practicing integrative medicine. Both groups were vying for that position and despite several meetings earlier in the year, could not come to an agreement.

My experience with WHI gatherings had shown me the possibility for understanding to develop between competing professionals, like a naturopath and a doctor. This could be amplified many times if each person in the room initially met on common ground. To this end, any meeting I conducted within WHI would commence with everyone having the chance to say something briefly, for example, about their day's highlight or why they'd come along. Even if it was just, 'Hello, my name's Bruce. I got my washing done today.' Bruce would no longer be invisible, as so many people can be at meetings. Importantly, with everyone's attention, albeit briefly, Bruce would also feel welcomed and encouraged to contribute to the group. Depending on the nature of the meeting this opportunity to speak would be limited to a stated time of say, no more than 30 seconds. Each person could also choose to pass on this opportunity if they so wished. Meetings were so much more productive following this formula.

I was curious as to whether this principle would work in such a high-powered setting and I took considerable time reflecting upon and finding a question that would hopefully bring each participant onto common ground.

The meeting was to take place on a Saturday. Once again Tori pointed out my need to rest each weekend and encouraged me to relinquish my role as chairman. In hindsight, I was inexperienced as to the amount of energy I would expend in such a daunting role. Unable or unwilling to see how vulnerable my health had become and convinced of the importance of the meeting, I went ahead.

Forty doctors flew into Melbourne from all states in Australia, each aligned to one group or the other. We sat in a large circle in the ballroom of an old Toorak mansion, named Armagh. Winter sunshine illuminated the garden outside the window as I began with a brief welcome and a grounding meditation. I then explained the approach we were going to take - to discover common ground first, so that the group as a whole would be more likely to achieve a wise decision.

While most of the practitioners in the room had spent many years in clinical practice, I wanted to take us all back to first principles, so I unleashed what I hoped would be the unifying question. I began by asking each person in turn to introduce themselves and briefly share: *Why they became involved in complementary medicine as part of their medical practice*, a choice that would potentially bring them into conflict with medical authorities. Their story would need to be contained within five minutes or less, with Mark Donohue seated to my left holding a silver bell, the designated timer.

One by one, each doctor was heard in turn, many utilizing their full allotted time, some in tears. Most of their stories related to personal or family health crises, many were heartrending and uplifting. It turned out, as I'd hoped, to be a moving process, connecting all of us in the room on a human level, regardless of affiliations.

At the morning tea break several doctors cornered me. Questioning my strategy, they asked me when we were going to get on with the 'real business.' When we re-gathered, I told everyone I'd been asked this question. Hoping like blazes I knew what I was doing, I paused, then said with some gravity, "For those of you wondering when we are going to get onto the 'real' business, this IS the Real Business!"

The sharing of individual stories continued until it came to a natural end by lunchtime. The rest of the day involved respectful discussion but ended without an agreed resolution. I knew I was in trouble!

Whilst many in the room were appreciative of the way I'd run the meeting, some were critical, especially when I called the meeting to a close as some members had to leave to catch flights. Those who were critical of what they perceived to be excessive 'Kumbaya' wanted to continue until a resolution was reached but I'd stipulated at the beginning of the day, and all had agreed, that when one person had to leave the meeting circle, the meeting would end. Besides which, I'd done as much as I was able to do, it was 5:00 p.m. and I was completely spent.

The critics need not have worried, within two weeks a phone discussion had ensued between Dr Kotsirilos and Dr Donahue in which the latter conceded that all things considered, AIMA was in the best position to play the role with the government (a role they still play). All was settled with the type of honest discussion modelled in the meeting.

I, on the other hand, had something to worry about. It reminded me of a slogan I once saw on a T-shirt: 'Elvis is dead, Sinatra too and me, I don't feel so good.'

The Plug is Pulled

From my perspective the day had been rewarding but very taxing. I struggled even more to get through the next two weeks at work, culminating in an event that turned my life 180 degrees. It took place on July 17, 1996. Sitting at my desk at the University finishing some paperwork, I was feeling tired but content. As coordinator of our department's fourth year teaching program, I was pleased that it was now completed for another year. My workload for the rest of the year would be a little easier for it. It was after 5:00 p.m. and most of my colleagues had gone home and I was about to follow them.

Without warning, I felt as if someone had pulled an energy socket out of the left side of my upper abdomen. (This sudden onset is not uncommon with Chronic Fatigue Syndrome (ME/CFS)) I was overwhelmed with extreme exhaustion and knew instinctively that something was seriously awry. I'm not sure how I managed to drive myself home that evening but when I arrived there, I told Tori I was unwell, collapsed into bed and slept for the next 18 hours only to wake up unrefreshed with my mind racing.

The fatigue reminded me of the experience I'd had in my 20's when I'd suffered from glandular fever (mononucleosis). I'd had anxiety and panic attacks sporadically in the past too but hadn't experienced these since I'd taken up regular meditation nine years before.

While I'd previously had the capacity to juggle many roles at once, it now took all my concentrated effort to hold a single role, even just briefly. I was also finding after periods of standing for any length of time that I would become dizzy and need to lie down. Much later, I would discover the reason for this; a commonly associated autonomic nervous system problem with ME/CFS is orthostatic hypotension, a drop in blood pressure that can be delayed for up to 10 minutes after sitting or standing upright, so that one frequently needs to lie down or risks fainting (the original 'Yellow Wiggle', Greg Page, was unable to work because of this problem). (See Orthostatic Intolerance subheading in Chapter 3)

Regardless of my own understanding at the time, it became apparent I needed a significant break away from work, simply because I could no longer do it.

It's a strange and frightening thing, one moment you're travelling along managing all the things you do in your life, next moment you've crossed an invisible line and your previous capacities are gone. Of course, I'd had four years of deteriorating health leading up to this moment and yet there was a clear breaking point. I sought help from numerous medical and alternative practitioners, but all my tests were normal.

It was as if an unseen protective bubble had burst leaving me vulnerable to the emotional elements. I'd always had the capacity to empathize and had an idea of what others were feeling, but now this was magnified to such an extent that it was like a tsunami. My meditation practice became difficult and when attempting to counsel someone with panic disorder I could no longer separate their panic from my own. Noisy, busy places, like shopping centres, became unbearable. My natural instinct was to seek retreat.

Professor John Murtagh, my university boss, was understanding having seen others with ME/CFS over his distinguished General Practice career and intimated that it might take me years to recover. So, once I'd organized coverage for my work roles, he allowed me to take my accrued sick leave, none of which I'd used up until then in my 8 years as a University lecturer.

It took seven weeks to either cancel or cover my various responsibilities. To give you an idea of what I was juggling at the time, here is a list (it makes me wobbly reading it even now!):

University - teaching 1st, 2nd, 4th and 6th year students and administrative responsibilities.

Clinical work - two four-hour sessions of predominantly counselling general practice work per week. Many of my patients had chronic illnesses with poor prognoses and they would come to see me for one or two consultations to have some hope restored, an irony I would reflect upon much later but sadly missed by me at the time! I was also a regular facilitator - 90 minutes one night per week for six weeks - of mindfulness-meditation courses, for groups of up to 10 people in the clinic where I was working.

[Note: When I first joined the University in 1989 for 12 months, I was also working a 19-hour shift once per week at the Knox Private Hospital covering their Emergency Department overnight.]

Public Speaking - Grand Rounds, conferences (e.g. I was invited to speak at the World Yoga conference in Sydney later that year) and WHI events.

Stress Management Consultancy - my regular clients included: Melbourne Airport air traffic controllers, six high schools for both students and teachers, careers counsellors and health practitioners of various persuasions.

The Whole Health Institute (WHI) - At its peak, WHI had a membership of over 640 people Australia-wide. We put on annual events including: a conference for the general public (I first met Tori at the 1991 conference); a doctor's conference; a student conference for health students of all persuasions; and various one-off speaker events. We published a directory of members and the Healing Currents Journal. All conferences included speakers, workshops, healthy catering and entertainment (Tori and I were part of a fun troupe of WHI comedy skit performers). We also had a regular one-hour community radio slot to fill each week. Meetings included a monthly Melbourne core group gathering and a quarterly board meeting.

There was only one paid member of the organization, our administrator, whom I met with at least weekly. We received no government funding or advertising income and relied entirely on membership and event participant payments.

Whilst we had a board of directors and various subcommittees, the overseeing and direction of all these activities was done by me. I was a passionate enthusiast but dreadful at delegation and did not protect my time with boundaries, so late-night phone calls were the norm. I loved the organization, the people in it and what it stood for, but the truth was I was working virtually a full-time voluntary job, on top of the rest of my work, and had fallen into the trap of believing I was indispensable.

As I relinquished my various jobs the most taxing and yet the hardest to let go of was my role as WHI president. Paradoxically, when I did, it was with a big sigh of relief.

Heading Rural

When you can no longer trust your body to cope with situations you previously found easy to deal with, everyday life becomes a challenge, especially in a city full of cars and noise. Post-exertional malaise (PEM) meant crashes into flu-like fatigue for days after minimal overexertion, physical and/or emotional. It could strike quite quickly or be delayed by a day or two. Some days I would be less fatigued, giving hope that I was turning the corner, but whatever energy I had would rapidly dissipate, often with minimal exertion, leaving me with my unwanted friend, overwhelming fatigue, once again.

Convinced I needed a long break to allow my body and mind to recover, Tori and I sold our Melbourne apartment, traded in our city car for a second-hand Subaru and went on a three-month camping/driving sojourn around Australia together. Tori was having struggles of her own at the time and didn't need much encouragement.

Vice president of WHI, Shirley Winter, and her husband Doug, lived in Perth, Western Australia (WA). They kindly offered for us to housesit and for Tori to do a locum job in their chiropractic clinic while they travelled overseas for six weeks. So, we had a destination.

With three months to get there we took a slow 4000km road tour through Australia. The trip with its simple lifestyle in connection with nature's beauty, early nights and no screens to watch, along with the friendly people we met along the way, restored some of my physical stamina.

At this time, I labelled what had happened to me as a 'burnout.' I was more than a little embarrassed that such a fate had befallen me, a meditation and stress management teacher. Over time it became clear that what was happening to me was a lot more complex than this. Along with my treating doctors, I was bewildered and unable to pinpoint or explain exactly what was going on. This contributed to a growing misunderstanding between me and our families. Finding out I fulfilled the criteria (see Appendix 1) for Chronic Fatigue Syndrome (ME/CFS) only magnified this.[1] In those days it was known as 'Yuppie Flu,' implying it was an illness of the middle to upper classes and implicating the person with the problem as the cause of their 'fake' disease and of staying ill. As you'll discover as you read on, nothing could be further from the reality of this terrible condition, which occurs equally across the population be you wealthy or poor.

After Perth, we moved to the Southwest of WA where we also had friends from WHI. We rented a rural house overlooking a 20-acre wetland in a town called Vasse, between the townships of Busselton and Dunsborough. Wetland birds and kangaroos were welcome visitors, while tiger snakes were less so!

Tori rented a room in a physiotherapy practice in Busselton, where she worked as a chiropractor. For our sanity we turned to creative pursuits; Tori drawing and painting, me writing and wild-life photography. All the while I tried many different modalities to improve my health: antidepressants, counselling, diets (the *Zone Diet* being the most helpful at that time), vitamins, herbs, body work, massage, energy healing. At one time I had acupuncture twice weekly for six months. Improvement was minimal.

I fell into a deep depression during this 14-month period, as I began to uncover some of the patterns from my childhood family dynamics that had contributed to my driven personality. I went into this dark pit willingly, as I believed that I had to go through it rather than around it and that maybe it would hold the key to my recovery. I'm sure a number of kangaroos were left traumatized by my screams!

Both my parents were Romanian Jews and survivors of the Holocaust. They arrived as teenagers in the late 1940's and built a life from scratch. They gave their all for their three children. Yet I would discover in the ensuing years that their childhood traumas were unwittingly, epigenetically or otherwise, passed on. The impact on children of Holocaust survivors, the so-called 'second-generation,' is deep and significant and I was no exception.[2] I would later receive invaluable assistance with this from a Jewish psychiatrist who had written a chapter in a book about his own experience as a second-generation child of survivors.[3]

Whilst 80% of ME/CFS follows a viral illness, a not uncommon antecedent that predisposes some (like myself) to this disease is childhood trauma. Whether this sets up a vulnerability in the immune system is yet to be determined.

After two years of living in WA, we moved back to our home state of Victoria. I hadn't recovered as quickly as I had expected to, so I was keen to continue living in a less stressful environment. We chose Apollo Bay, a favorite destination from both our childhood and rented a farmhouse overlooking the town. Tori saw clients from home, before moving her business into a natural therapy clinic in town. It was a beautiful place to live and being part of a small community (permanent population of 900) was a rich and unique experience.

Highlights included the characters we met, being part of the community choir and participating in an amateur theatre production. This said, our seven years there were some of our most challenging. I badly injured my back, chopping wood. I lost 10 kg in weight over our first winter. The weather was too often cold and misty for our liking and getting out of town meant at least 45 minutes of driving through winding mountain or coastal roads, an exhausting proposition. As my need for health services beyond the town increased, this became problematic.

My efforts at creating alternative work and income were also thwarted. A junior novel I wrote, inspired by my nephew Andrew, failed to find a publisher, despite some promising leads. A poster series I created from my photographs taken of wildlife in Vasse, attracted great interest but no distributor. Frustratingly, I lacked the strength and energy to promote these ventures myself as each push led to days of push-back PEM and lots of expletives!

As my illness and inability to work dragged on for years on end, like so many people affected by ME/CFS, I heard the whispers: 'not really sick,' 'a malingerer,' 'a retiree,' 'just depressed,' and no doubt some other less voluble choice descriptions!

I saw a documentary once, about a type of seabird, the male of the species with red stripes on its beak. The female birds and the bird community generally were most impressed with the male with the most 'red stripes.' I don't believe we humans differ too greatly from this. As a financially secure, successful doctor, I had lots of metaphorical 'red stripes.' Unable to work, on a disability pension and renting, with the unsexy label of ME/CFS, my red stripes had faded to grey. My salvation was, not in Tori's eyes.

Chapter 5

ME/CFS UNMASKED?

"Whenever a new discovery is reported in the scientific world, they say first, "It is probably not true." Thereafter, when the truth of the new proposition has been demonstrated beyond question, they say, "Yes, it may be true, but it is not important." Finally, when sufficient time has elapsed to fully evidence its importance, they say, "Yes, surely it is important, but it is no longer new."

MICHEL DE MONTAIGNE (1533-1592)

Yes, "It IS all in your head!"

At the base of the brain lies the brainstem. Through a hole in the skull, it connects to the spinal cord which communicates via nerves with the rest of our body. The brainstem is pivotal in regulating the unconscious functions of our bodies. In fact, it is the body's life-support system. It contains the nerve-centers of what is called the autonomic nervous system (ANS). The ANS plays many roles and it performs these behind the scenes, without us even thinking. This includes; maintaining appropriate heart rate, blood pressure and body temperature. It also keeps us breathing, digesting, pooing and transitioning from being awake to being asleep. The ANS is also the center for the fight or flight (stress) response.

A more recent discovery is that it performs an important role in modulating our immune system and muscle metabolism, where energy production is so critical. Given its diverse influence upon so many body systems, could the brainstem be one of the linchpin causation sites in ME/CFS?

43

Physical Evidence: Craniocervical Instability (CCI) mimics ME/CFS

Jeff Wood and Jennifer Brea had been diagnosed with severe ME/CFS. Both turned out to have Cranio-cervical Instability (CCI). Their stories are compelling and make for fascinating reading see https://www.mechanicalbasis.org/. CCI probably makes up a very small proportion of the people diagnosed with severe ME/CFS, nonetheless it may give us a clue as to the mechanism behind the wide range of symptoms we see.

CCI is more common in conditions like Rheumatoid Arthritis, Ehlers Danlos and Downs Syndrome. Ehlers Danlos syndrome affects the connective tissues supporting bones, skin, blood vessels and organs. People with this syndrome often exhibit extremely loose and flexible joints and if this occurs in the vertebrae at the top of the neck the brainstem becomes vulnerable to compression which leads to inflammation and subsequent malfunction. Similar problems can exist in Down Syndrome.

Yet neither Jeff nor Jen had these other Syndromes and why such a serious skeletal problem would become apparent at this time in Jeff and Jen's lives is unclear. Both began with a viral-like illness, typical of ME/CFS and their symptoms were ME/CFS-like and included post exertional malaise (PEM), autonomic nervous system dysfunction with heart rate and blood pressure abnormalities, including Postural Orthostatic Tachycardia Syndrome (POTS) and brain fog. They appeared to have a severe version of ME/CFS.

Importantly, **unlike** ME/CFS, CCI can be treated both non-surgically and surgically. This includes cervical traction, strengthening exercises and physical therapies or via the route eventually taken by Jeff and Jen, major cervical fusion surgery with three months in hospital. What I find fascinating here is that both Jeff and Jen found that **all** of their previous ME/CFS-like symptoms, including post-exertional malaise

(PEM) were gone when the pressure was taken off their brainstem by this surgery and the compressed brainstem had time to recover!

Before Jeff had definitive surgery to his cervical spine, he had what is called a Halo Brace placed around his head. Before it had been tightened sufficiently to relieve the compression on his brainstem, Jeff was able to use his hands to lift the brace himself and therefore in real time experience the effects of decompression. He gives this intriguing description:

"For the past four years, ever since the onset of my severe ME and POTS, my standing heart rate was usually in the 130's or higher. But, with maximum halo lift, this suddenly didn't seem to be the case. I felt so different—I suddenly felt... kind of healthy? I grabbed my pulse ox (Jeff had bought a medical grade pulse oximeter) and measured. Sure enough, my standing heart rate was 86! I couldn't believe it. This seemed too good to be true, and I couldn't accept this so easily. I had to verify this was actually happening. So, I let go of the halo, and my skull sank downward. My heart rate measured 127. I lifted the halo again with maximal traction, and my heart rate was now 82."[1] He repeated measurements with the same result every time, making the surgeons decision to go ahead with major decompression surgery an easy one.

Their extraordinary stories raise many questions like:

- While CCI is still considered relatively rare, is there a small proportion of the people diagnosed with ME/CFS that actually have CCI?
- Could the initiating illness/trigger have somehow (for example via an autoimmune phenomena) weakened the ligaments in the upper cervical spine?
- Does this physical example (i.e. CCI) of a neurological problem with identical symptoms to ME/CFS help confirm that neuroinflammation generally is the primary source/driver of symptoms in ME/CFS?

- Critically it raises the need to be thoroughly assessed to exclude causes other than ME/CFS before concluding it is ME/CFS. Remember, ME/CFS is a diagnosis of exclusion (See Appendices 1 & 2), Jeff and Jen had CCI and therefore by definition did NOT have ME/CFS.

Brain Inflammation

There are now half a dozen positron emission tomography (PET) brain imaging research studies looking at the brains of people with ME/CFS. PET scans detect levels of a molecule called translocator protein whose level rises in the presence of neuroinflammation. Consistently these PET scans have demonstrated neuro-inflammation in widespread brain areas, most commonly affecting the brainstem in people affected by ME/CFS versus healthy controls.[2,3] In addition to this, other brain scanning techniques have shown more white matter (the 'connecting wires' between brain cells i.e. grey matter) in the prefrontal cortex of people with ME/CFS.[4]

It is postulated that this increase in white matter might occur as a corrective response to brainstem inflammation which has effectively, temporarily at least, damaged the lines of communication from, to and through the brainstem. The brain, in an attempt to correct this blockage builds more wires (i.e. white matter).[5]

Another research review paper has pointed out some similarities between ME/CFS and Multiple Sclerosis (MS).[6] Fatigue and post-exertional malaise are shared by both illnesses, along with pathological changes indicated by neuro-inflammatory markers and mitochondrial (energy producing 'batteries' within all cells) dysfunction. Poorly functioning mitochondria is now a recognized feature of several neurological conditions.

By contrast, brain scans of the brains of people with MS demonstrate a reduction of white matter rather than an increase as seen in the scans of people with ME/CFS. Of further interest is that Diffusion Tensor Imaging MRI (DTI) scans of individuals with depression reveal measurable decreases in white matter integrity, not the increased amount of white matter evident in people with ME/CFS. The DTI results showed that the participants with depression had reduced white matter integrity when compared with the participants without depression.[7]

The researcher's conclusion was as follows: *"Thus, although anxiety, depression and ME/CFS may share (some) biological similarities, on the present evidence, ME/CFS appears to be a distinct disorder.*[8]*"*

Of further significance, the level of abnormality on the researched brain PET scans corresponded with the clinical level of severity of the person with ME/CFS. This brings hope that brain PET scans may be used in future to more accurately diagnose and grade the severity of ME/CFS.

Mucus 101

A biology update: Mucus lines our respiratory, gastrointestinal and in women, genital tracts. It protects us against invaders, be they viruses, bacteria, fungi, parasites or toxins. It also works in harmony with our microbiome, healthy bugs that coexist and line these tracts working with the mucus to help protect us against unhealthy invaders. Hence, having defective mucus proteins can be a serious issue. We know this from its role in other diseases like Crohn's disease in the gut and Sjogren's Syndrome that dries out skin, mouth, eyes etc.

We also know that people with ME/CFS and other neurological diseases lack the same diversity of healthy microbiome bugs in their gut when compared with healthy people and that this can allow the entry of harmful pathogens and toxins (a Leaky Gut Syndrome).

Many viruses enter our bodies via the upper respiratory tract, especially the common cold virus, a member of the coronavirus family. They enter via the nose and travel to the rear of the nasal passage. Here, they are hopefully beaten back. But if they penetrate the mucus barrier, they can enter the brain through a thin area of skull-bone known as the cribriform plate. On the other side of this plate lies the Olfactory nerve, the nerve that carries our sense of smell.

In susceptible people with 'weakened' mucus, viruses, the most common triggers of ME/CFS, could potentially gain access to the brain causing a firing from our next line of defense, white blood cells, who release pro-inflammatory cytokines. These cytokines in damaging the invader may inadvertently cause the brain inflammation evident on brain PET scans.

Interestingly, one of the first symptoms in some people who catch COVID-19 is loss of the sense of smell. Could those with this symptom be more likely to develop ME/CFS? We don't yet know, but what we do know is cases of long-COVID illness are not uncommon as people recover from the acute illness only to find themselves in a new battle. We'll explore this further in Chapter 7.

Genetic Predisposition - The 'nose' has it?

So often these days we hear people talk about how our genetic codes predispose us to this disease or that. As Cort Johnson, from the website *Health Rising*, so succinctly puts it, "there are alterations in genes and then there are ALTERATIONS. Most small genetic changes make little or no difference. Others dramatically change the functioning of the protein they produce.[9]"

When Travis Craddock and his fellow researchers at Nova Southeastern University in Florida, recently compared genes relating to mucus proteins, our first line of defense against pathogens and toxins, he found an ALTERATION.[10] In around 80 % of people with ME/CFS compared with close to 0% of healthy people's genes, there was about as deleterious a genetic alteration as you can get, an alteration suggested by previous research[11,12] but not detected until now.

They found people with this defective gene produce a puny, truncated, likely dysfunctional protein that is a third the size of normal. This mucous protein known as Mucous 19 protein forms the outer gel layer of the mucous which prevents toxins, pathogens, and irritants from getting to the skin layer where the nerves are. Note, the number 19 in its delineation (Mucous 19 protein), is incidental and bears no relation to the '19' in the name COVID 19 but could be very important in its acquisition as we will see below.

Craddock speculated whether a dysfunctional mucous layer might be contributing to neuroinflammation in ME/CFS. He proposed that the compromised gel layer could result in an altered microbiota (normally healthy bugs) in the nose. This lack of adequate protection could irritate the nasal membranes, so that a chronic low grade non-allergic inflammatory response would result. The irritated nerves beneath the skin could also produce the increased sensitivity to chemicals often seen in ME/CFS.

Craddock noted that a weakened mucous layer could also allow pathogens, toxins and other compounds entry into the blood (Leaky Nose Syndrome?) producing a systemic reaction which flares up other ME/CFS symptoms such as the better-known Leaky Gut Syndrome might do.[13]

COVID-19 Entry

As yet, I'm unaware of research looking at the weakened nasal mucus (Mucous 19 protein) increasing susceptibility to COVID-19 or those people with this weakness subsequently being more vulnerable to post-

Covid illnesses, like lung fibrosis or ME/CFS, but as you'll see, it may be very significant.

Recent research has identified two specific nose cell types as likely initial infection points for COVID-19. Scientists discovered that mucous producing goblet cells along with ciliated cells (which help sweep the mucus along) were chock-full of the entry proteins that the COVID-19 virus uses to get into our cells. This readily available surface entry point within our noses could help explain the high rate of transmission.

The study with Human Cell Atlas Lung Biological Network found cells in the eye and some other organs also contain the viral-entry proteins. It's possible that future research may uncover the weakened protective mucus 19 protein genetic variant as also playing a role in allowing this virus easier entry in those more susceptible. Watch this space.

Gulf War Illness

Gulf War Illness (GWI), is a multi-symptom chronic illness occurring in around 250,000 of the 697,000 US Veterans exposed to chemical toxins in their deployment in the Persian Gulf War of 1990-91.[14,15] It is almost identical to ME/CFS in its presentation. Over the past 25 years the vast majority of soldiers with this condition have remained unwell, despite the fact that they were young men fit for duty prior to deployment in 1990.

A recent PET Brain scan comparative study looked at 23 veterans, of whom 15 had GWI, eight veterans without GWI and 25 healthy civilians. The scans detected little evidence of neuroinflammation in the healthy controls and veterans who were free of GWI. By contrast, the study found extensive inflammation in the brains of veterans with GWI, "particularly in the cortical regions, which are involved in 'higher-order' functions, such as memory, concentration and reasoning," says Zeynab Alshelh, PhD, one of two research fellows who co-led the study. "The neuroinflammation looked very similar to the widespread cortical inflammation we detected in Fibromyalgia patients (in earlier studies)," says Alshelh.[16]

It supports the fact that chemical exposures can be an onset trigger for some people with ME/CFS. A secondary school teacher in her forties who'd consulted me for her ME/CFS put the onset down to exposure to an industrial detergent that was accidently being used nearby at 200 times the recommended concentration.

If you are interested in learning more about the anatomy and function of the brain generally, the following link is a good place to start - https://www.healthline.com/human-body-maps/brain#brain-diagram

If you are interested in looking further at the research into neuro-inflammation and ME/CFS, the following link introduces Jarred Younger (PhD), a leading researcher in this area - https://www.healthrising.org/blog/2015/07/15/the-neuroinflammation-man-jarred-younger-on-inflammation-fibromyalgia-and-chronic-fatigue-syndrome/

Chapter 5
Key Points

- ✓ The brainstem is located within the base of the skull and connects with the spinal cord.
- ✓ It contains the Autonomic Nervous System (ANS), which in a well person maintains heart rate, breathing, blood pressure, gut function, body temperature, the stress response and the transition from awake to sleep.
- ✓ ANS malfunction within the brainstem can produce all ME/CFS symptoms as seen in Cervico-cranial Instability CCI.

✓ CCI can lead to brainstem compression triggering ANS malfunction and therefore mimicking ME/CFS. It is an important differential diagnosis as it can be treated with specific rehabilitation and/or surgery.

✓ Unlike ME/CFS, CCI can be treated surgically with excellent outcomes possible.

✓ PET brain scans not only confirm the presence of brainstem and cortical inflammation in people with ME/CFS but can also predict the severity of their illness on scan alone.

✓ The pattern of increased white matter on MRI scans of people with ME/CFS differs from MS, anxiety and depression and confirms its status (on scanning) as a unique neurological phenomenon.

✓ Pathogens, such as viruses, may enter the body via the nose or gut and trigger the inflammation in the brainstem.

✓ Gulf War Illness (GWI), which has many similarities to ME/CFS, and also has as yet no cure, was triggered by toxic chemical exposure, and brain scans of afflicted soldiers and people with Fibromyalgia, provide further evidence that neuroinflammation appears to be the source of symptoms in both conditions.

Chapter 6

TRIGGERS

"Shields are down, divert all energy to life-supports."

CAPTAIN KATHRYN JANEWAY, STAR TREK VOYAGER

How it Begins

In most illnesses of a chronic nature, an individual's genetic code plays a role and ME/CFS is no exception. This has been identified in problems with immune function where specific patterns of genetic expression have been located.[1,2] The importance of genetic factors is confirmed by the fact that ME/CFS is significantly more common in identical twins (55% concordance) than non-identical twins (19% concordance).[3-6]

Apart from the association with certain genetic markers in people with ME/CFS, there is also a more common history of childhood trauma than in the general population.[7] These factors can predispose the body to be more vulnerable to stressors, such as viruses, that can trigger the onset of ME/CFS (See Fig 1).

Often prior events that weaken the immune system can become triggers later down the track. For example, it is thought that if a person has exposure to a mold toxin, their body may store the toxin in particular cells, generally fat cells, in order to protect the rest of the body. This can be due to genetic factors weakening their body's detoxification systems, making it unable to eliminate the mold toxin completely. If, years later, further mold toxin exposure occurs when the body has no more storage room, multiple systems become vulnerable and the person is tipped into ME/CFS as a result.

Another possible antecedent example would be a persistent virus which lies dormant. For instance, one of my patients recovered from Infectious Mononucleosis (caused by the Epstein Barr Virus (EBV)), after three difficult months when she was 22. Her genetics/epigenetics – I'll explain later - was such that the virus was not completely eliminated and thus lay dormant. It reactivated 10 years later at a time when her body was under the strain of other stressors, like being over-worked and sleep deprived. This time around it resulted in her developing ME/CFS. There are some who theorize that reactivation of latent viruses is the likely mechanism for most with ME/CFS.[8]

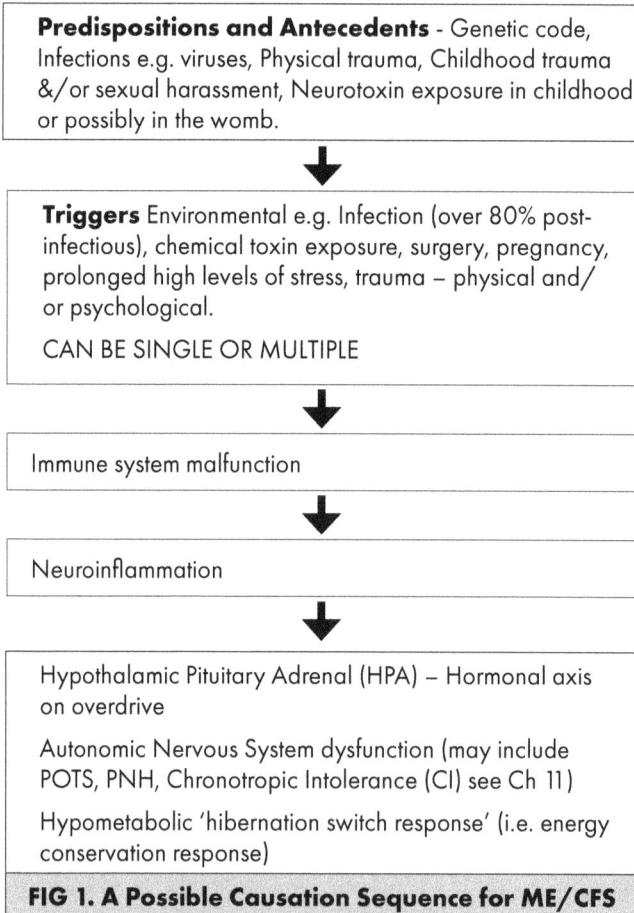

Predispositions and Antecedents - Genetic code, Infections e.g. viruses, Physical trauma, Childhood trauma &/or sexual harassment, Neurotoxin exposure in childhood or possibly in the womb.

↓

Triggers Environmental e.g. Infection (over 80% post-infectious), chemical toxin exposure, surgery, pregnancy, prolonged high levels of stress, trauma – physical and/or psychological.

CAN BE SINGLE OR MULTIPLE

↓

Immune system malfunction

↓

Neuroinflammation

↓

Hypothalamic Pituitary Adrenal (HPA) – Hormonal axis on overdrive

Autonomic Nervous System dysfunction (may include POTS, PNH, Chronotropic Intolerance (CI) see Ch 11)

Hypometabolic 'hibernation switch response' (i.e. energy conservation response)

FIG 1. A Possible Causation Sequence for ME/CFS

Infectious Triggers

While brainstem compression and exposure to neurotoxins, as we explored in Chapter 6, can be triggers for the onset of ME/CFS, they are not considered the most common triggers. Infections are, with viruses the most common of all. In over 80% of cases, viruses such as Epstein Barr (EBV), influenza virus, Cytomegalovirus (CMV), entero (gastro) viruses, Human herpes viruses (HH6, HH7) are implicated as known triggers.[9] The SARS CoV-1 virus,[10,11] that caused the 2003 SARS epidemic, the precursor to our current pandemic virus SARS-CoV-2, triggered ME/CFS (we'll look at this more closely in the next chapter). Other infectious triggers implicated include the zoonotic bacterium, *Coxiella Burnetii (Q Fever) and* the parasite, giardia.[12]

It is thought that in vulnerable individuals the body's immune response is faulty. Its attempts to kill the infectious agent may cause collateral damage, leading to the brain-inflammation and dysfunction as we explored in Chapter 5, with all the symptoms of ME/CFS that ensue. (see Fig 2).[13-16]

The Dubbo Study

The prospective Dubbo study in 2006 supports this model.[17] Dubbo is a rural town in New South Wales, Australia, with a surrounding population (in 2006) within a 200 km radius of 104,000. There were 253 volunteers (all over 16 years of age) who presented to their GPs with acute viral-like symptoms including fatigue of less than 6 weeks duration. They had blood tests and were followed up over a 12-month period.

Test results indicated acute Glandular Fever (EBV) in 68 people, Ross River Virus (a mosquito-borne virus common in this region) in 60 people and Q Fever (Coxiella Burnetti - a type of bacteria) in 43 people. In a further 82 people with an infection neither of these three diagnoses were made, so the infectious agent was not identified, presumed to be viral.

At 6 months follow up there were 29 people still unwell with 28 (11% of the recruited 253), of these fulfilling the diagnostic criteria for ME/CFS. The number one predictor of whether their illness persisted beyond 6 months was the **severity of the acute illness** regardless of the specific infective trigger. Notably neither demographic (age, sex, level of education, whether employed or not) or psychological factors predicted whether the person would go on to develop ME/CFS.[18]

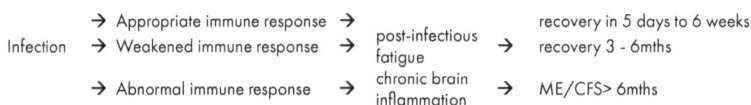

	→ Appropriate immune response →		recovery in 5 days to 6 weeks
Infection	→ Weakened immune response →	post-infectious fatigue →	recovery 3 - 6mths
	→ Abnormal immune response →	chronic brain inflammation →	ME/CFS> 6mths

FIGURE 2 The Infectious Cascade to ME/CFS

In some people, ME/CFS can follow on from a single triggering event, as Chris demonstrated (see p.14-5) when contracting EBV (Infectious Mononucleosis). In others, like myself (see Chapter 4) a series of illnesses and/or stressors precedes the final collapse into exhaustion with all the other wretched symptoms.

It is possible there are many different subtypes of illnesses contained within the banner of ME/CFS, the identification of which may help to focus our management strategies further in future.

The International Research Symposium on ME/CFS that Tori and I attended in March 2019, concluded that we are dealing with a neuroimmune multisystem disease with typical patterns. I will elaborate on this shortly. At the symposium it was also postulated that the severe form of ME/CFS, which leaves people housebound and often bedbound, may be a different illness to the milder or more moderate versions of the illness.[19] Researchers and treating practitioners in this area need to be mindful of this possibility, but this said, my experience with people with ME/CFS seeking my assistance, is that a gentle rehab approach, which we will explore in some detail in *A Path Back to Life,* is safe regardless of the severity of the illness. The key, as I discovered in my own life-restoration, is starting where you are at, pacing and building very slowly and mindfully from there.

In a Nutshell ?

One possible way of conceiving how this all fits together is that predisposing factors, like genetics, toxin exposure, infection and/ or childhood trauma set the body up to respond inappropriately to triggers later in life. A healthy person would have an acute appropriate overdrive response to such triggers, before their body systems reset back to normal drive. In a person predisposed to ME/CFS their body systems go into and remain in overdrive, as well as becoming more sensitive to further triggers, which perpetuates the problem.

Eventually, for reasons not yet fully understood, the body switches to an energy conservation 'hibernation' response, a low energy state which expresses itself in a common pattern (regardless of the initial cause) of exhaustion and the myriad of problematic symptoms associated with ME/CFS as described in Appendix 1. So, while there may be different triggers in different people affected by ME/CFS, these roads converge into a common recognizable pattern of symptoms, many of which appear to result from brainstem inflammation. In *A Path Back to Life* we'll look at ways that can return the body to a healthier state.

Chapter 6
Key Points

- ✓ ME/CFS onset can follow single or multiple triggering events.
- ✓ Genetic predisposition and antecedents, such as viral illnesses, toxin exposure and trauma (physical/ psychological or both) can make one vulnerable to developing ME/CFS.
- ✓ Triggers are often the same as or build upon the antecedents. In over 80% of cases a viral infection is the trigger.
- ✓ The Dubbo Study found around 11% of people who experience a significant viral illness, such as EBV or RRV (Ross River Virus) will go on to develop ME/CFS, with the severity of the acute illness being the strongest predictor of it becoming chronic.
- ✓ Ultimately, regardless of the initial trigger, their appears to be a brainstem switch to a energy conservation 'hibernation response,' leading to a typical set of ME/ CFS symptoms.
- ✓ There is growing evidence that COVID-19 will soon trigger a pandemic of ME/CFS and we'll hone-in on the evidence for that in the next chapter.

Chapter 7

LONG COVID – THE GROWING WAVE

"There are many steps clinicians can take now to improve the health, function, and quality of life of people with ME/CFS, including those newly ill with ME/CFS following COVID-19. This guidance may also help Long COVID patients, even if they do not fully meet criteria for ME/CFS."

DR LUCINDA BATEMAN - MYALGIC ENCEPHALOMYELITIS/CHRONIC FATIGUE SYNDROME: ESSENTIALS OF DIAGNOSIS AND MANAGEMENT. MAYO CLINIC PROCEEDINGS CONSENSUS RECOMMENDATIONS. 25TH AUGUST 2021[1]

The COVID-19 pandemic is leaving much of the world's population devastated in its wake. First wave, second wave, third…plus new strains emerging around the globe has left millions of loved-one's lost, and as if all this isn't enough, it's become apparent there's a slower more insidious wave rising in its wake.[2] There is genuine concern that the chronic effects of this coronavirus will be ongoing in many of those who've been infected, including some younger people with what seemed originally to be a mild version of COVID-19.

Things are changing rapidly, currently as I type, we are experiencing the Omicron variant that unlike previous strains tends to attack the upper airway rather the than the lungs. Even as you read this the information will be out of date. Nonetheless, since its onset in 2019, a variety of different variants have already set in train a trail of chronic illness. In fact, it's estimated **the number of cases of ME/CFS will double world-wide following the COVID pandemic.**[3] Let me explain.

As we discussed in the previous chapter, lingering symptoms including fatigue can follow various types of infectious illnesses. These "post-infectious" fatigue syndromes resemble ME/CFS. Moreover, ME/CFS is known to most commonly be triggered by viral illnesses, including coronaviruses. When viral disease symptoms stretch out beyond their usual length of time the illness is initially labelled 'post-viral.' At this stage I'd suggest you could easily rename these as 'long-Epstein Barr virus (EBV or Mononucleosis), 'long-Cytomegalovirus (CMV)', 'long-Ross River Fever (RRV)' and yes, 'long-COVID'. However, recall that if the debilitating effects extend beyond **three months in children or six months in adults** and include the other criteria in Appendix 1, then all these labels would converge into the one diagnosis: ME/CFS.

What's In a Name?

To clarify, while the acute potentially life-threatening illness is called COVID-19 (short for Coronavirus Disease 2019, as the first recorded case was in 2019), the coronavirus causing it is officially named SARS-CoV-2. Long-COVID, can occur after the acute illness and is also known by the following names: post-COVID, long-haul COVID, post-acute COVID-19, long-term effects of COVID, or chronic COVID.[4]

Given the checkered history ME/CFS has (see Chapter 2), not surprisingly people with long- COVID do not want to be labelled in this way. In fact, even the proposed label of Chronic Covid Syndrome (CCS), which can be broken down to various sublabels depending on the predominance of symptoms. E.g., Chronic neuro-Covid or Chronic respiratory-Covid etc., is proving to be unpopular.[5]

Why label at all? The short answer is so researchers world-wide can clarify their investigations from the same definitions and clinicians can be clearer on their prescriptions. Sounds reasonable and it is. But as my story attests in the next chapter, ME/CFS has not been respected as a legitimate disease, despite the terrible levels of debility it can inflict. In addition, a 'Syndrome' is not taken as seriously as a 'Disease', and this is reflected in the relatively miserly funding that has been provided for ME/CFS research in the past.

Long-COVID people do not want to be treated in this way, hence the resistance to any association with ME/CFS or CCS. While this is entirely understandable, it would, I believe, be a foolish mistake to ignore research and wisdom hard-won. People with long-COVID need not reinvent decades of experience but take advantage of the lessons from research and clinical treatment experience gained from managing ME/CFS.[6]

Whilst it's true there is no specific cure as yet for ME/CFS, this, as I've said, is a rapidly evolving area of research around the world. Rehab understanding is a part of this and the changing the terrain strategies outlined in *ME/CFS – A Path Back to Life* and the Mayo clinic recommendations[7] suggest, have the potential to be as invaluable for people with long-COVID as they've been for people with ME/CFS, many of whom, with steady application, have been able to return to at least part-time work as I've done. Make no mistake, appropriately individually prescribed paced rehabilitation strategies can make the difference to being bed or housebound, disabled, or active once more in the community.[8,9]

COVID'S Course

Like ME/CFS patients, those with long-COVID conditions have recounted being dismissed by health care professionals.[10] So let's dispel this nonsense and review what we know about the different routes COVID can take.

While most people with acute COVID-19 get better within weeks of illness, around 10% go on to experience long-COVID conditions.[11] **Long-COVID conditions** include a wide range of new, returning, or ongoing health problems which may be experienced **four or more weeks** after first being infected with SARS-CoV-2. Yes, this means even people who never had COVID-19 symptoms could, in the days or weeks after they were infected develop long-COVID conditions seemingly out of the blue! We don't have enough information yet to know if this applies to the Omicron strain or future variants of concern.

These long-COVID conditions can involve different types and combinations of health problems for different lengths of time from weeks to months. Unlike some of the other types of long-COVID problems that only tend to occur in people who have had severe illness (we'll touch on these in a moment), these symptoms can happen to anyone who has had COVID-19, even if the illness was mild, or if they had no initial symptoms, this is particularly so for those who are unvaccinated or were infected prior to vaccines becoming available. The Center for Disease Control (CDC) in the US reports various combinations of the following symptoms can occur with long COVID:[12]

- Difficulty breathing or shortness of breath
- Tiredness or fatigue
- Symptoms that get worse after physical or mental activities
- Difficulty thinking or concentrating (sometimes referred to as "brain fog")
- Cough
- Chest or stomach pain
- Headache
- Fast-beating or pounding heart (also known as heart palpitations)
- Joint or muscle pain
- Pins-and-needles feeling
- Diarrhea
- Sleep problems
- Fever
- Dizziness on standing (light-headedness)
- Rash

- Mood changes
- Change in smell or taste
- Changes in period cycles

If you check this list against Appendix 1, you'll note ME/CFS presents similarly. A study of patients still **ill 6 months** after mild or moderate acute COVID-19 found that **about half met criteria for ME/CFS,**[13] effectively shifting the diagnosis from long-COVID to ME/CFS in those 50%.

As mentioned in the introduction to this chapter, this will likely lead to a doubling of cases of ME/CFS world-wide with massive implications for individuals, family, health care systems, society and economies.

Some of the COVID "long haulers" may have symptoms reflecting organ damage, such as to the lungs or heart, from the acute disease.[14] Other long haulers also display similar symptoms but have no clear evidence of such organ damage.[15] Clearly it will be necessary to distinguish these two groups as each may require different treatments. Let's explore this further.

Multiorgan Effects of Severe COVID-19

Some people who've had severe illness with COVID-19 experience multiorgan effects or autoimmune conditions with symptoms lasting weeks or months after the acute COVID-19 illness. Multiorgan effects can affect most, if not all, body systems, including heart, lung, kidney, skin, and brain functions. Autoimmune conditions happen when your immune system attacks healthy cells in your body by mistake, causing inflammation (painful swelling) or tissue damage in the affected parts of the body.[16]

If a person with COVID-19's health is deteriorating (e.g. worsening breathlessness, dizziness, disorientation) then they may need hospitalization, which can be life-saving but can also leave its own mark in terms of complications.

COVID-19 Illness and Hospitalization

Post-intensive care syndrome (PICS), refers to the physical, cognitive and psychological changes that occur after surviving any serious illness or injury that requires ventilation treatment in the ICU. These health effects that begin when a person is in an intensive care unit (ICU) can remain after a person returns home. These effects can include severe weakness, problems with thinking and judgment, and post-traumatic stress disorder (PTSD). PTSD involves long-term reactions to any very stressful event.

Some symptoms that can occur after hospitalization are similar to some of the symptoms that people with initially mild or no symptoms may experience many weeks after COVID-19. It can be difficult to know whether they are caused by the effects of hospitalization, the long-term effects of the virus, or a combination of both. These conditions might also be complicated by other effects related to the COVID-19 pandemic, including mental health effects from isolation, negative economic situations, and lack of access to healthcare for managing underlying conditions. These factors can affect both people post ICU who have experienced COVID-19 and those who have not.

It's worth noting, on average, if a person with severe COVID-19 requires an ICU ventilator machine to assist their breathing they will need this assisted ventilation on average for around three weeks. This may change as treatments improve and variants of concern become more or less dangerous. The Omicron variant and vaccination availability have already reduced the chances of ending up on a ventilator. But regardless, if you do this is still likely to be many times longer than the three to four-day average of non-COVID patients needing ICU ventilation.[17] This takes a huge toll on the body, a person's mental state, not to mention a country's health care system, many of which are ill-equipped for the large numbers needing ICU, let alone the length of ventilator time requirement keeping the bed occupied. It is worth noting that while treatments continue to improve, currently, less than a third of the ventilated COVID-19 cases come off the ventilator and survive.[18]

These survivors will also be the most at risk of developing long-COVID complications. I've listed all of the currently known long-COVID illnesses in Table 1.[19-25]

Lifestyle Prevention of COVID

It is early days to answer the question of what makes one person infected with COVID more vulnerable to go on to develop a long-COVID complication with any certainty but we do know a little. The unvaccinated; frail people over 60 years of age; and those living in deprived circumstances are more vulnerable to developing serious sequelae with acute COVID as well to develop long-COVID.[26]

Lifestyle is also important. People with obesity, for instance, are more likely to end up with more severe COVID. This risk is compounded if they have the co-morbitities of diabetes and/or cardiovascular disease. See:

https://www.obesityevidencehub.org.au/collections/impacts/impact-of-obesity-on-covid-19-outcomes

A fascinating study of over 1000 health care workers published in the British Medical Journal demonstrated the power of diet on minimizing COVID's impact.[27] It looked specifically at those working in high risk COVID environments in six different countries. While diet did not prevent COVID infection or alter its duration if contracted, those who ate a predominantly plant-based or plant-based and fish diet were more likely to have milder versions of COVID if they contracted the disease. By contrast those on low carbohydrate/high protein diets were more prone to developing severe COVID.[28]

We'll explore the potential role of diet in managing ME/CFS in some detail in *A Path Back to Life*.

- Neurological (inflammation and/or degeneration)
  - Dysosmia/parosmia/loss of ability to smell and taste
  - Long-COVID (Post-viral Syndrome < 6 months)
  - ME/CFS (> 6 months)
  - Stroke
  - Guillain-Barre Syndrome
  - Parkinson's Disease (increased vulnerability)
- Post Intensive Care Syndrome (PICS) – (if recovered after being on a ventilator in ICU)
- Post Traumatic Stress Disorder (PTSD)
- Multiple organ damage – can affect all major body organs, including lungs, heart, brain, kidneys and immune system inflicting in some, permanent damage e.g. lung fibrosis with reduced lung capacity by up to 30%; myocarditis/cardiomyopathy.
- Multisystem Inflammatory Syndrome (MIS) – rare and most commonly occurs in children during acute COVID or later

TABLE 1 Identified COVID-19 Long-term Complications[19-25]

Long Haulers

Despite the conclusion of the Dubbo study[29] (see Chapter 6) that the severity of the acute infection rather than the virus type was most predictive of whether people went on to develop ME/CFS, it appears that all COVID-19 survivors are at risk of these additional complications, regardless of the severity of the initial illness.[30]

As we now know, it's not just the oldies who are in danger either. In the first US wave former Governor of New York, Andrew Cuomo, noted that over 50% of the people hospitalized in New York City with COVID-19 were aged between 18 and 49 years.[31] The Delta and

Omicron variants of COVID have shown a propensity to infect the young, **especially those unvaccinated.**

This is a novel virus i.e. before 2019 it had never been seen by any of our immune systems. So, while unvaccinated older people are more likely to die of this virus because their immune systems tend to be less sharp in their response as they age, young people are not invulnerable to longer term complications. They may be much less likely to die of COVID but are vulnerable to serious long-term complications, some of which, like ME/CFS, can be debilitating and life-long.[32]

Dr Fauci's 2020 Observations

In a July 2020 interview, Dr Anthony Fauci, America's top infectious diseases specialist charged with guiding the US response to COVID-19 was one of the first to officially acknowledge the likely link with ME/CFS. "If you look anecdotally," he said, there is no question that there are a considerable number of individuals who have a post-viral syndrome that really in many respects can incapacitate them for weeks and weeks following so-called recovery and clearing of the virus.... you can see people who've recovered who really do not get back to normal and that they have things that are highly suggestive of myalgic encephalomyelitis and chronic fatigue syndrome. Brain fog, fatigue, and difficulty in concentrating, so this is something we really need to seriously look at because it very well might be a post-viral syndrome associated with COVID-19."[33,34]

SARS-CoV-1: A 2003 Precedent

Though not widely publicized, there has been a precedent for this. What came to be known simply as SARS (Severe Acute Respiratory Syndrome) was caused by a related coronavirus in 2003. It was officially named SARS-CoV-1.

This 2003 outbreak was a far smaller pandemic than COVID-19 but when considering deaths per infection, SARS-CoV-1 was even less forgiving than its related CoV-2. It infected around 8000 people in 29 different countries and had a 10% fatality rate, around 10-times more deadly than the original SARS-Cov-2 strain. Fortunately, SARS-CoV-1 was nowhere near as infectious as SARS-CoV-2, allowing it to be corralled so that it did not go onto become a more widespread pandemic. In some of those who were infected and survived, however, it inflicted similar long-term effects to the ones we're seeing now.[35]

Long SARS CoV-1 _ The Research

A 2003 study of a SARS-CoV-1 outbreak in Canada involving 345 people who'd tested positive, found 44 had died of the virus while **12 months later 17% of the 301 survivors** continued to **be too unwell to work at all**. An additional 9% were unable to return to full-time work. The reason for these 26% (17+ 9) of survivors struggling to work was being sick with ME/CFS-like symptoms.[36]

Another study of a SARS-CoV-1 outbreak in Hong Kong followed up 55 people with an average age of 44yrs (27 were Health Care Workers (HCW)) who'd survived.[37] They followed and tested their health status over a two-year period. They concluded: "Two years after SARS onset, more than 50% of this highly selected group of SARS survivors had impairment in DLCO (a measure of lung function). Their exercise capacity and health status were remarkably lower than that of the general population and 30% of these HCW's had not returned to work. SARS can lead to persistent mental and physical abnormalities in survivors, with a greater adverse impact on HCW's. Health authorities should provide good support and follow up for these patients including HCW's."[38]

Further longer-term follow-up research of people who survived SARS-CoV-1 reported in 2011 by Harvey Moldofsky and John Patcai at the University of Toronto in Canada, described 22 people with SARS, all of whom remained unable to work 13–36 months after infection[39] Compared with matched controls, they had persistent fatigue, muscle pain, depression and disrupted sleep. Another study,[40] published in 2009, tracked people with SARS for 4 years and found that 40% had chronic fatigue. Many were unemployed and had experienced social stigmatization.

Can SARS Help Now?

While development of a SARS vaccine in 2003 was being investigated, this research was discontinued when SARS-CoV-1 was contained with the sort of measures we're using today i.e. social distancing, face masks, hand washing, PPE etc. However, recently it has been reported that people who were infected and yet recovered from SARS-CoV-1 who have now received an m-RNA COVID-19 vaccine have mounted a much more robust healthy immune response than most people. Even stronger than those infected for a second time with SARS-CoV-2 or after receiving any of our current COVID vaccines without pre-exposure to SARS-CoV-1. **In other words, the best immune responders for Cov-2 were those infected with CoV-1 in 2003 who subsequently had an m-RNA CoV-2 vaccine.**

This is leading scientists to re-examine the SARS- CoV-1 virus to see if they can develop even more effective vaccines against CoV-2 (COVID 19) by incorporating some of the CoV-1 antigens (e.g. slightly different spike proteins) into updated COVID vaccines.[41]

Epidemiologist with Long-COVID

In the August 13, 2020 edition of journal *Nature*,[42] Nisreen Alwan, an Associate Professor of Public Health at the University of Southampton, UK, gave this description of her ongoing struggles with COVID:

"I had COVID symptoms of fever, cough, gastrointestinal upset, chest and leg pains in late March...Since then, I have had bad days with some symptoms, then OK days, then worse days of exhaustion, making me regret what I did on the OK days, such as taking a short walk." Descriptions like this are typical of post-viral fatigue that can follow on from numerous different viruses (see previous chapter). As I've said, if these symptoms persist for 6 or more months, they would most likely fulfill the criteria for ME/CFS.

Dr Alwan continues, "This is a difficult time for me as a public-health academic engaged in pandemic action while struggling with this strange pattern of illness. I don't know what it means for my long-term health, which is concerning as a mother caring for young children. One consolation is knowing that I am not alone. There are many others who have not regained their previous health, even months after their initial symptoms. Among them, fluctuating symptoms like mine are common."

Relapsing and Remitting Course

The fluctuation in symptoms can be confusing to those unfamiliar with ME/CFS. What is most likely is the ME/CFS relapses that can emanate post COVID-19, just like other viruses, will be linked to over-exertion (mental or physical) and demonstrate features of the individual's initial illness minus the fever.[43,44] So if you started with a sore throat and fatigue or a cough and fatigue, or breathlessness, then these are the likely symptoms, together with all the other typical symptoms of ME/CFS (i.e. Unrefreshing sleep, brain fog, poor concentration etc.), to be prominent during a flare up of long-COVID ME/CFS.

We now know that this waxing and waning of symptoms is common in neurological diseases. Multiple Sclerosis (MS) is an example of a disease, like ME/CFS, that was labelled as hysterical 60 years ago for this very reason before people identified the pattern and the underlying neurological pathology was identified. Let's not make the same mistake with long-COVID.

Permanent (Non-fluctuating) Symptoms?

As discussed earlier, unlike other viruses that can lead to ME/CFS with its fluctuating symptoms, such as, Mononucleosis caused by the Epstin Barr Virus (EBV), with long-COVID-19 there seems to be another layer of non-fluctuating symptoms that occur in some. This can be due to permanent fibrosis (scarring) in the lungs or inflammatory disease within blood vessels, the heart, kidney, immune system and brain (see Table 1). In addition, animal research and the pattern of cellular defense suggests an increased vulnerability to the degenerative brain disease Parkinson's disease (PD), which, like COVID-19 often also commences with a loss of the ability to smell.[45]

Even before COVID-19, it had been proposed that PD could be the result of an autoimmune post-viral syndrome.[46] We know viruses can cause neurological disorders like ME/CFS, Polio and Post-polio Syndrome being an example. The Influenza A pandemic of 1918/19 has also been linked to Encephalomyelitis Lethargica, a neurological disorder portrayed in the feature film *Awakenings*.[47] Again, time and more research is needed to clarify if COVID-19 increases the chances of developing PD.

How Many Become Long Haulers?

Many researchers are now launching follow-up studies of people who have been infected with SARS-CoV-2. Several of these focus on damage to specific organs or systems; others plan to track a range of effects. In the United Kingdom, the Post-Hospitalisation COVID-19 Study (PHOSP-COVID see https://www.phosp.org/) aims to follow 10,000 patients for a year, analysing clinical factors such as blood tests and scans, and collecting data on biomarkers. A similar study of hundreds of people over 2 years was launched in the United States at the end of July (see https://www.nature.com/articles/d41586-020-02598-6).

A smaller Australian study at St Vincent's Hospital in Sydney has been following 78 people who developed COVID 19 and has found two months after the initial infection 40% are still unwell. This study will continue to follow up for at least 12 months.[48]

The most common long-term effect of COVID-19 is its least understood: severe fatigue. This said, as I presented in Chapter 5, inflammation in the brainstem is likely the cause and SARS CoV-2 has been demonstrated to cause inflammation in numerous sites within the brain.

See https://www.news-medical.net/news/20201217/Study-shows-an-inflammatory-response-in-the-mice-brain-is-responsible-for-severe-COVID-19.aspx

Increasing numbers of people have reported crippling exhaustion and malaise after having the virus. Support groups on sites such as Facebook host thousands of members, who sometimes call themselves "long-haulers". They struggle to get out of bed, or to work for more than a few minutes or hours at a time. One study of 143 people with COVID-19 discharged from a hospital in Rome found that 53% had reported fatigue and 43% had shortness of breath an average of 2 months after their symptoms started.[49] A study of patients in China showed that 25% had abnormal lung function after 3 months, and that 16% were still fatigued.[50]

A recent report in the British Medical Journal found one in seven children infected with COVID still had symptoms 15 weeks later.[51]

A Real Time Study

One fascinating current study is being undertaken by the Open Medicine Foundation (OMF). OMF is a US research organization studying ME/CFS.[52] In this particular $1 million dollar research study, they are taking blood samples from the general population and following those who develop COVID with further blood testing, measuring immune system biomarkers and seeing which people go onto develop long-COVID in the form of ME/CFS, hoping to find clues as to the antecedent determinants of being susceptible to ME/CFS generally. This knowledge may lead to new treatments.

COVID Vaccine May Help

With the COVID-19 vaccination rollout around the globe there have been some surprising reports. For instance, some COVID-19 long haulers with ME/CFS symptoms for over 8 months reported significant improvements in their symptoms immediately following vaccination or within two weeks of the first shot of the vaccine.

How many? Some surveys of the symptoms of long haulers who'd received the vaccine found around 1 in 20 had completely returned to normal, while around 1 in 25, had reported a significant worsening of symptoms.[53] The rest of those surveyed fell somewhere in between, with a positive effect of the vaccination on symptoms pipping a negative affect overall.

More recent research has shown the vaccine **reduces the risk of developing long-COVID by 50% in the double vaccinated.** https://www.bbc.com/news/health-58410[54]

More long-term research is needed. However, what we know already does open up our minds to further possibilities for immune system modifying treatments for ME/CFS such as vaccines for COVID and other viruses linked with triggering ME/CFS.

Summing Up

New research is arising daily into COVID-19 and long–Covid. So, watch this space. Unfortunately, I can only conclude from the available data at this stage that it seems at least 10 to 30% of people who develop COVID-19 will go on to develop long-COVID and this will be yet another huge challenge that humanity is going to have to face with this pandemic.

As a recent feature NEWS article in Nature concludes, "The answers will not come quickly. The problem is, to assess long-term consequences, the only thing you need is time." See https://www.nature.com/articles/d41586-020-02598-6

With millions of people worldwide developing long-COVID post viral fatigue and many of these continuing on as the even 'longer' ME/CFS, the implications for those suffering and for society more broadly are mind-boggling and challenging.

In the next chapter we'll look at our own story (Tori and me) not only as a cautionary tale of what can happen when adequate validation and support is lacking, but what can be done when it is given. Now we know the truth about ME/CFS, a truth ironically that thanks to long-COVID-19 will become more real by the day, we need to embrace rather than recoil in ignorant disbelief from those who'll be falling through the medical cracks, unable to simply get up and carry on, and provide them with the support they'll need to have a fighting chance at life-restoration.

One day we may have an immune modifying cure for post viral syndromes like long-COVID and ME/CFS but as we do not yet have these specific treatments, it is imperative to reduce the impact of this wave of cases by introducing ME/CFS-specific rehabilitation measures, such as pacing, finding the balance between not pushing through and not stopping all together, and the early adoption of the other strategies I've outlined in some detail in *ME/CFS - A Path Back to Life*. We've witnessed in our clinic as have others in theirs, how these simple measures can help diminish the level of debility and the duration of the ongoing illness seen in ME/CFS. It can be done.

Chapter 7
Key Points

✓ In the current pandemic of COVID-19 it is estimated at least 10% will go on to develop long-COVID with some going on to be defined as ME/CFS.

✓ In regions/countries experiencing high numbers of COVID-19 cases like the UK, US, Brazil and Europe, it is likely that a significant rolling wave of ME/CFS will follow.

✓ SARS-CoV-1 in 2003 had a high level of ongoing serious debility, leaving many unable to return to work.

✓ Ongoing complications following acute COVID-19 recovery, already include post-Intensive Care Syndrome (PICS), permanent lung damage, cardiomyopathy and post-viral fatigue (COVID) Syndrome and the beginnings of an ME/CFS wave.

✓ If SARS-CoV-1 is anything to go by then given the millions of people infected with SARS-CoV-2, even once we all receive a vaccine (a wonderful thing for those of us who were never infected), there will still be chronic ill-health impacts left behind, with all of the personal, social and economic implications for most with long-COVID.

✓ Current estimates are that COVID -19 vaccines will prevent 50% of further cases of long-COVID. They also may contribute clues as to how to treat ME/CFS via vaccination immune system modification in future.

✓ It appears for a small percentage of the COVID long haulers the COVID-19 vaccine may turn out to be a surprising cure. However, most will be presented with the challenge of long-term rehabilitation.

✓ Experience with ME/CFS has shown whilst no specific treatments have been discovered, there are general measures (which require some careful explanation) that I outline in some detail in *ME/CFS- A Path Back to Life* which can minimize the chances of downward spiraling debility and maximize the chances of significant improvement or recovery.

Chapter 8

MY EXPERIENCE/CESSATION OF FAMILIAR SUPPORT (ME/CFS)

"To have ME/CFS is to experience hell twice over, firstly through the devastation of the disease itself, and secondly through the lack of diagnosis, information and support that most sufferers are still having to endure."

CLARE FRANCIS, ME/CFS PATIENT AND BEST-SELLING AUTHOR

With no definitive test to make the diagnosis, it is little wonder that people with ME/CFS, like Clare (quoted above over 20 years ago!),[1] still frequently express feeling damaged by the response of treating doctors and their closest family and friends, when for months and often years their struggles are 'not being believed.'[2,3]

In 1988 the prestigious journal, Science, concluded that having a lack of emotional support in your life was a greater risk factor for disease and death than smoking.[4] This came on the back of research that demonstrated the most lonely and isolated had 3 to 4 times the risk of dying prematurely when compared with those with close social ties.[5,6] To appreciate the magnitude of this, consider the fact that those with close social ties and unhealthy lifestyles (such as smoking, obesity and lack of exercise) actually lived longer than those with poor social ties but more healthy living habits.[7] It is therefore of great significance if a chronic illness, like ME/CFS, leads to increased social isolation.

Research has uncovered that people with ME/CFS are indeed less likely to have good social supports than healthy people.[8] This is not surprising given debility leads to social isolation. It is a double-edged blade, however, because treatment of ME/CFS is less likely to succeed if there is poor social support.[9,10]

In my clinic I observed that adolescents still living at home had a better chance of recovery. They had no bills to pay or work obligations and their parents, seeing the reality of how the illness had affected their child, could not deny its seriousness. The months or years needed to bring about recovery could usually be incorporated into the family dynamic. In contrast, older people with ME/CFS were often met with disbelief and struggled to achieve the support they needed to tackle the illness.

Validity and Support

For some people, like myself, ME/CFS not only brings social dysfunction but significant loss of career and independence. For others it can mean the complete breakdown of their marriage or family ties.

As you'll see in Tori's description of me in the next Chapter (Ch 9), people with ME/CFS have lost the ability to function in areas of life healthy people take for granted. Just getting through a day showered and fed can be a major challenge that many cannot manage alone.

For example, for those people rendered housebound by ME/CFS, research has shown that the measure of disability experienced can be equal to the disability experienced by people undergoing chemotherapy for cancer, or with other chronic conditions, such as AIDS, multiple sclerosis, end-stage renal disease and chronic obstructive pulmonary disease.[11] And yet, as I've shared with my own story and Chris's story (see Chapter 1), it can attract little or no sympathy or support from family or friends and even members of the medical profession.

Just as in mental illnesses,[12] the lack of obvious physical abnormalities; we can often look well enough, can contribute to this attitude. Plus, in Australia at least, people with this condition have until recently been unable to access a disability support pension or funding from the National Disability Insurance Scheme. This is now changing yet is still a ridiculously demanding application process for people to endure who are so unwell.

This lack of validity, understanding and emotional/financial support, in people desperately in need of these things, can remove all opportunity for recovery. Remember too that ME/CFS patients are highly motivated (in clear distinction from severe depression that is characterized by reduced motivation), willing to do just about anything to get well, and frustrated by not being physically able to function anymore; a far cry from the 'lazy' archetype they may have been painted with. The illness simply has them trapped.

Mental Health and ME/CFS

Despite all our new understanding of this illness, the echo of 'Hysteria' (See Chapter 2) still remains an issue. So, what does the research tell us? The incidence of reduced mental health after the onset of ME/CFS is similar to that experienced in other chronic medical conditions, yet better than that seen in depression.[13,14] The prevalence of depression and anxiety in ME/CFS is similar to that in other disabling, chronic illnesses.[15,16] It's tough being that sick and depression and anxiety will occur in many, but they are **not the cause of the illness**.

A heads up here, telling someone with ME/CFS you know how it feels because you feel sad and tired at times, is a bit like telling a person who has had their arm chopped off that you understand how they feel because you've experienced a paper cut!

Both from personal experience and from observing my patients with ME/CFS, I've come to understand 2nd Generation Holocaust survivor and author Eva Hoffman's insights into suffering, when she says, "And it may be that suffering shared, suffering respected, is suffering endurable. Suffering that is misunderstood or dishonored can turn on the self in unendurable pain."[17] Feeling guilty or ashamed for having this illness and not being able to 'will' yourself out of it, can also lead to depression or worse.

Compounding this situation of not being heard or understood can be the reaction the person with ME/CFS makes to this bizarre lack of recognition of their daily challenges. Commonly they will feel a need to tell everyone who will listen about their many symptoms. A problem shared is a problem halved may be true enough but be careful who you share it with! The effect of this on people who do not believe you have a real illness anyway, is to further reinforce their belief that you are in fact a hypochondriac. Ultimately this leads to the character of the person with ME/CFS in some way being seen as 'deficient' or 'weak', 'bringing this all upon themselves,' in effect a character assassination. My own experience of this led me to suicidal despair.

Turning of the Backs

I've experienced no deeper pain than that of having the people I thought loved and cared for me, turn their backs on me. We simply don't appreciate the power of our personal community (family, friends and acquaintances), which provides us with the unseen social glue that supports and holds us together every minute of the day, until it is diminished or gone. This has been a huge awakener for me.

One day, I found myself looking in the mirror and trying to reassure myself, saying, 'but it's me, why am I being treated so differently? I'm still here! I just have this terrible illness.' My mental health was severely challenged as it was, with the loss of my career, friendships, sense of purpose and financial security. I was a high achieving, motivated person who loved his job, I would never have consciously chosen to put myself in this situation.

I found myself reeling for days after difficult conversations where people I once trusted treated me like I was a fraud; Tori was on suicide watch for years. In the end, reluctantly in a way, for I longed to be part of the social glue that had supported me when I was well – but to preserve my life and get my head back above the quicksand, I had to stay away from negative inputs as much as possible, including family, and surround myself with friends who believed in me and my ability to find a way to overcome this illness. To this end Tori and I are forever grateful to our fabulous GP's, Dr Denise Ruth and Dr Aurelio ('Joe') Di Stefano and our very special friends who stuck with us.

I have since observed that some healthy people with a lack of personal experience of chronic illness, just 'don't do illness.' That is to say, they find it difficult to genuinely empathize or be with a person with a chronic disability. Whether this is due to their genetics determining an emotional limitation, or a lack of experience and not knowing what to say, or simply because they are deeply fearful of it themselves and don't want any reminder that they too might be vulnerable, I can merely speculate. Whatever their reasons, they are emotionally unsafe people to be around if you're feeling at all fragile and not people you want with you in the trenches of life.

Of course, any chronic illness can bring out the worst in a person's personality and I was certainly guilty of this at times. Anyone living with a loved one experiencing chronic pain will testify to this. In this situation the illness or injury causing the pain is quite correctly attributed to be the factor that changes the person's personality. This is very different from concluding, as many people ignorant of ME/CFS do, that their changed personality IS the illness.

Financial woes

When both our families misunderstood and rejected our situation in 2002, it corresponded with a time in our lives of deep financial strife. After protracted stressful appeals, that ended in the Federal Court, we were ordered by the court to pay $50,000 tax on a lump sum income insurance payout I'd eventually received in 1999. The Federal tax law upon which this judgement was made was recognized as unfair and changed the year after! This lump sum was derived from an Income Protection Policy that was meant to cover me until the age of 65. I'd had to accept cancellation of my policy for a small payout as ME/CFS was an unacceptable diagnosis to the insurance company, and it was a case of take the lump sum or end up with nothing.

I was a proud young man with a strong and successful work ethic. The lump sum and cashing out my superannuation on hardship grounds had staved off having to face Centrelink (Social Security). Now, unable to provide for us and Tori struggling with her mental health I saw all the relevant health practitioners, filled in the copious forms and was eventually placed on a Disability Support Pension (DSP).

I felt the full weight of embarrassment and shame this represented in my own and our families' minds. My GP at the time, an ex-work colleague from Monash Uni, Denise, bless her, wept openly during a consultation we had with her when Tori and I shared our predicament.

Without her help and that of another dear friend, Judy, a very intuitive and compassionate person, I seriously doubt I would have survived. Judy, upon hearing my despair over the phone, dropped everything and drove three hours from Melbourne to spend time with me. In the late 1980's, Judy had introduced me to the Whole Health Institute (that I had become President of (see Ch 4)).

While Tori worked, Judy drove me to a wonderful lookout amongst the Mountain Ash trees in the nearby Otway hinterland behind Apollo Bay. We opened the windows and breathed in the forest air. We had not spoken in depth for years, but I've discovered, with the best of friends, the gate can easily be reopened.

"Right!" Judy said, "tell me from the beginning, I want to hear it all, especially the cringy bits!" Over the next four hours I poured out my sorry tale. As we sat, we could see the ocean relentlessly pounding the cliffs far below. The house Tori and I were renting had a second story and Tori was afraid I would leap from the upstairs balcony, but in my own disturbed mind, these cliffs were my escape hatch; walking distance from home (on a good day!), I could throw myself off and let the ocean clean up the mess. In my mind I'd made enough of a mess of our lives trying to 'save the world' and the last thing I'd want was to leave yet another mess for Tori to clean up. [These are some of the typical thoughts and distorted logic of someone in deep depression. This is not normal. If you are having feelings of worthlessness, like this, share this with someone you trust, like your GP or call Lifeline.]

Judy listened, listened and listened some more…until finally the words dried up, and tears began to fall. She placed her arm on my shoulder as I wept and wept. "It's not your fault and you're not crazy," she said. More tears. Another car pulled up at the lookout next to us. My tears dried up.

"Let's step outside and stretch a little," Judy said.

We walked a short way as she confided that another good friend of hers, Bev, who'd had ME/CFS for eight years, had a similar story of being a successful health professional yet was now unable to work. "At least you have Tori," she said, "Bev's husband has left her and no one in her immediate family believes her… She lives alone now in a caravan park barely surviving on a pension."

Judy fired up. "Like you, Bev is a decent, caring person who loved her work. And, what? Suddenly she's a malingerer! It stinks!" She continued, "ME/CFS is real alright. It's a societal blind spot and your families' interpretation is the problem," she said. "Regardless, suffering is suffering. Neither Bev nor you should need to justify that!"

We drove back down to the coastline and met up with Tori for a meal back home. We joked around sharing funny stories from our past before Judy had to leave. "Hang in there, guys!" she said, "there'll be a flipside to all this, you'll see." We had a group hug. Soon after I fell into a deep sleep as Judy drove back to Melbourne.

Children

Tori and I shared our feelings and thoughts regularly, yet there was one huge issue that we could not agree upon. Without our immediate families' emotional support, in my depressed debilitative state along with our precarious financial position I'd let go of us having children as a real possibility. Tori, on the other hand, with her biological clock ticking, desperately wanted kids.

In our courtship we'd talked about having two or three kids and how much we were both looking forward to parenting. Yet, life doesn't always go as planned! Within 18 months of our marriage, I'd become seriously ill and now 6 years later, I felt like an abject failure. We were facing bankruptcy and I couldn't get off the couch!

Tori continued to work as a Chiropractor and care for me but was clearly burning out and struggling with her own depression. As the pressure built so did the volume of our 'discussions'. Each time the word children was mentioned, or I even saw a child I'd feel my fragile self-esteem implode into a spiral of inadequacy... and those cliffs beckoned.

We were maxed out on our credit cards and it felt like our world was falling apart. Every time I pushed myself to help out more, I would be struck down by Post Exertional Malaise, sometimes for weeks leaving Tori with even more work to do. It was so FRUSTRATING!

At one point, I pleaded with Tori to leave me and find someone else. I knew how badly she wanted to be a mum and I didn't think it was fair for her to spend her life nursing me. We both knew that on my own, my options were limited. In terms of government assisted care, I'd be placed in an Assisted Aged Care facility. No other alternatives existed for disabled forty-somethings as I was then.

The dead lock seemed impassable despite seeking help from counsellors. More years, more 'discussions' and more tears, until one day Tori looked into my eyes and said: "Stevie Sommer, I married you for better or for worse and I'm never going to leave you with or without children. If you try to run away, I'll catch you (she knew I couldn't run very fast!). Besides who's going to make me laugh?" she said. We wept and held each other tight. From that moment on those cliffs began to fade.

Grief Cycles

Loss is part of the cycle of life. While we might think we'd love to win and be happy all the time, in fact it is through loss and struggle that we grow. In order to deeply appreciate what's most important, we must learn to accept loss. In ME/CFS, opportunities to do this are writ large!

While different cultures and individuals may differ in the ways they express grief, it helps us to understand that grief is a normal life process and rather than fight it, to allow the feelings that arise to cycle through. Below are stages of grief as originally conceived by Elisabeth Kubler-Ross.[18,19] Next to each phase, I've put examples from my experience with ME/CFS.

Denial and Disbelief	e.g. "I'll be right after a few months of rest."
Fear, loss and worry	e.g. "I've lost my health and ability to work, promising career, income, many family members and friends. How will I/we survive?"
Frustration and anger	e.g. "Why can't I just do what I used to! I'm sick of crashing!!!"

Guilt	e.g. Leaving Tori to do everything. Not feeling able to start a family.
Sadness and Depression	e.g. See chat with Judy looking over ocean cliffs above.
Acceptance	e.g. "We may never be able to have kids, but we've got each other and maybe we can be foster parents one day."

Acceptance

ME/CFS patient Dean Anderson talks about what acceptance meant for him.[20] He believes that reaching a certain kind of acceptance was the key to his recovery. He described it not as resignation, but rather "an acceptance of the reality of the illness and of the need to lead a different kind of life, perhaps for the rest of my life." To him, acceptance also meant finding ways "to be productive and [to] find fulfillment under unfamiliar and difficult circumstances."

Like Dean, once I began to accept my situation and shift my focus from what I couldn't do, to what I could do, I was able to turn out to the world more and savor little things again. Like jokes, birdsong, sunshine sparkling on the water, a pigeon soaring on the breeze… I was also able to realize that while I might not be able to help much with physical tasks, I could still help Tori just by listening and helping her to problem solve.

Perhaps paradoxically, for ME/CFS patient Dean and me, this also seemed to open the door to recovery. For me ultimately this led to an understanding of the slow, patient, micro-rehab approach I share in some detail in *ME/CFS – A Path Back to Life.*

Roots, Scaffolding and Politics

It is important to note the holistic rehabilitation approach I took with my ME/CFS patients between 2007 and 2011 was not prescriptive. It provided principles and ways for individuals to make their own way back to better health as I did.

For this rehabilitation approach to work, however, it required a supportive environment, roots and scaffolding if you like, where people could feel safe and secure. Hence, if people with ME/CFS are to attempt to restore even a small amount of their previous capacities, it is of the utmost importance they can access adequate financial support for food, shelter and health care. As I've already noted, young people still at home may be able to access this via family. However, for people who do not have this support, who'd previously been working and living independently when struck down by ME/CFS, it can be a nightmare. Given our new understandings that have arisen from research worldwide, especially in the past five years, it's time that we as a community accept that ME/CFS is a chronic debilitating neurological disease deserving of our support and provide for peoples' needs via an appropriate safety net.

It is **important to note**, with the rehabilitation approach I am proposing, it is **not a quick fix**. It can take months and often years for people to return to a level of health where they can support themselves. Therefore, it does not negate the responsibility of the government or our society to assist people with ME/CFS to live more fully, as with any other debilitating condition that already attracts government assistance.

As I have pointed out many people with ME/CFS are more debilitated in their activities of daily living than people in virtually any other disease grouping that already attracts government assistance in the form of disability and insurance/pensions.

Even those who have a level of recovery may need to utilize skills, like pacing in the workplace, to manage their ongoing life, be it part time work or otherwise in a way their employer can understand and accept.

If government or insurance company assistance was based upon how well a person can function rather than a disease label, then we could better meet the needs of those people who need it most. The National Disability Insurance Scheme (NDIS) in Australia has recently taken up this functional model.

For now, whilst we don't have a straightforward diagnostic test such as a blood test for ME/CFS, Government departments overseeing pension payments could require a person with ME/CFS to obtain a diagnostic assessment from a GP who can verify the patient has been through all the current international standards of diagnostic testing. This could include, along with a relevant history and standard examination to exclude other conditions, (see Appendix 1 and 2), a 10-minute NASA Lean Test (Ch 3).

If governments are going to provide the appropriate supports, then society in general will need to accept the biomedical rather than psychiatric reality of ME/CFS, a reality accepted by the WHO. So, at the end of Chapter 12 I've summarized much of the research culminating in a summary table.

With this research understood along with the research on the levels of disability ME/CFS can bring, can I humbly suggest that government disability assistance be given to people with ME/CFS based upon their ability to function, which could be reviewed, for instance, annually, as improvement is possible. In Australia this model has been adopted by the NDIS.

Chapter 8
Key Points

✓ We are social beings and social support is always important, especially when we are unwell.

✓ Epidemiological research confirms that having a lack of social support is perhaps the biggest major risk factor to our health. Bigger than smoking and obesity combined.

✓ When we're sick, regardless of the illness, we need congruent validation for what we're experiencing to enhance our chance of improvement. For perhaps complex reasons, unlike many 'acceptably recognized' chronic illnesses, this validation has been lacking for people with ME/CFS. For too long now, despite ongoing research confirming it is a neurological multi-systems disease, ME/CFS has been lumped into the too hard box, rather than an admission of 'we don't know yet.' The **latest research suggests we do in fact know. (See Ch 10-12).**

✓ A lack of validation for one's suffering is one of the most painful experiences a human being can feel. For one experiencing ME/CFS it feels cruel and unfair to have to face both the illness and the rejection.

✓ Congruent support is the fundamental platform (roots and scaffolding) people with ME/CFS need in place to enable them to get a firm footing to pull themselves clear of the quicksand this disease inflicts. In this way they can begin to make steps towards getting well, a process which can take months or years.

✓ Research shows that people with ME/CFS have more chance of recovery if receiving validation and adequate support. This support may take the form of understanding family, friends, Support Groups (face to face or on-line) and health professionals familiar with or specializing in ME/CFS.

✓ There is now adequate research confirming ME/CFS as a biomedical neurological multisystem disease (see Chapters 10-12) and Government assistance based upon need is desperately required for many with this debilitating condition.

Chapter 9

A DAY IN THE LIFE – A CARER'S REFLECTION

BY TORI SOMMER

"Be kind to yourself."

TORI SOMMER

I crawled out of bed to switch off the alarm. Steve followed me, dragging himself out from under the covers to sit alongside me. He was hunched on the edge of the mattress with one hand stretched out behind me and the other gripping the bedhead for balance. Plumes of flattened bed-hair stood upright at the back of both our heads. He returned my grin faintly as I tried to settle his hair back into place.

'Sorry I kept you awake' he said, 'I couldn't sleep for quids and I'm sick of being in bed.'

A tinge of colour was draining from his face with the effort of sitting and he sank back down into bed again as I covered him with the doona. I had to get a move on to get ready for work but if he felt able to manage it, I could help him shower.

He was three days into a crash and felt absolutely wasted but couldn't bear to leave his hair unwashed any longer.

I hurriedly washed, dried and dressed, glanced at the time on my phone and dashed back to the bathroom to place the plastic chair in the shower recess and adjust the water temperature. Steve slowly clambered out of bed and on to his feet. He crept down the narrow hallway towards the bathroom, pressing his hands along the walls for support.

He slumped down onto the chair under the flow of water, and I washed his hair in silence, trying to avoid rivulets streaming down my forearms and dripping into my shoes. I had to make it brief but knew that rushing would only sap what precious little energy Steve had. So, I tried not to stress about running late for work by focusing on my breathing, to steadily get him washed, dried, and dressed before his energy waned altogether.

I left him to briefly soak in the warm, soothing stream while I raced to flick on the kettle in the kitchen.

As I waited for the water to boil, I glanced through our kitchen window across the foothills of the Otway ranges. The sea mist lingered in a snow-white sheath over the township below. Our farmhouse hovered above it, the sunshine spilling over the back deck, the gentle boom of ocean waves on Marengo reef trying to soothe my concerns. Surely a person with ME/CFS could heal in this place, I thought desperately?

I returned gripping two cups of herbal tea that I rested on the vanity then helped Steve from the shower, placing the chair in front of the basin so he could rest while I dried his hair. He sat down awkwardly and doubled over in pain as a wave of cramping struck.

Along with his fatigue and weight loss was a severe form of irritable bowel syndrome. As much as we loved the old weatherboard farmhouse we were renting, the dunny in the lean-to out the back was ramshackle and riddled with way too many spiders for our liking. The hallway and lean-to were also cold beyond the warmth of the bathroom; I needed to get Steve's thick hair dry and help him dress before he could use the toilet.

With the morning routine finally over, the couch was Steve's daily friend and he collapsed into it with relief. Lying there meant he wasn't bedbound, and he felt connected to the garden and sunlight through the loungeroom windows. The bookshelf was just beyond reach, so

I usually helped him select something for the day to read. He was a voracious reader by nature and thankfully could still accomplish this in small bursts. On a good day he had enough energy to read his medical books or journals and walk slowly to the mailbox at the front of our house and back. Today, the shower, especially with the hair wash would cost him his reading energy, but I made a pile of books beside the couch in hope.

As predicted, he closed his eyes in a quiet meditation instead.

I understood the signal. Talking required the little energy he had and was trying to conserve. His lymph glands were up again as was usual when the illness flared, and he was aching all over as though full of a nasty case of flu.

But I found it hard to be quiet today. Apart from the fact that Steve and I had so many interests in common and it was always enriching, even briefly, to delve into one topic or another together, there was a pressing concern I needed to talk about.

I resisted the urge to turn on the news or listen to music to distract myself while I prepared breakfast, knowing Steve's sensitivity to noise was so acute. I tried not to be noisy, carefully placing the bowls on the counter and trying not to rush and rattle the contents of the cutlery drawer as I searched for a spoon, but that was hard as I was already running late, as usual.

My first patient was due at my clinic in under two minutes, so I told Steve I'd be back to make us some lunch and left his bowl of muesli with lactose free milk, yoghurt and berries, some snacks, and another cup of tea on the side table next to his couch. I placed the landline telephone strategically on the floor at arms-length from where he was lying. He knew he could call me at work in a crisis. I felt relieved that he was settled for the morning, and just had to try for the time being to push aside my concerns over a recent phone call with my dad, Ian.

I felt a deep need for understanding and acceptance, especially from my father, to approve of Steven again as he had at the beginning of our union. With a pang of sadness, I recalled how he had given a delightful speech at our wedding several years beforehand and pinned a cheerful yellow badge on Steven's lapel that read, 'Very Special Person.'

As Steven's health and career faded, I sensed that in my father's estimation, so did the gloss on that badge. In fact, I was starting to feel that today Ian would now tear it from my husband's lapel, metaphorically speaking.

I opened the front door of the Natural Therapies Centre I shared as a chiropractor with a naturopath and masseuse. There I found my first little patient rolling a toy fire truck across the carpeted waiting room as his mother sat and waited. Five-year-old Felix swung the truck around as I entered, greeting me with a pretend shower of water from the fire hose and a high-pitched wail mocking the sounds of a siren. It was a fitting start to my day.

Pushing aside my own weariness, I focussed on treating my budding firey, followed by several other local families, the parish vicar, and some tourists. The morning ended with one of my favourite patients, the kind, warm hearted father of a friend and neighbour, an elderly gentleman and father of nine who was also a surviving war veteran and Rat of Tobruk.

Jack's old eyes glistened as he revealed how he'd endured one of the raids as a 17-year-old on the front line, by sheltering in a shallow pit in the ground as bombs rained down around him. He thought he would die but managed to survive one of the bloodiest conflicts on African soil in WW2.

Walking home via the fish co-op during my lunch break, I reflected on Jack's traumatic personal story and found it helped bring my own concerns into stark perspective. I suddenly felt childish in my own struggles for paternal acceptance and determined I should not raise the topic of my father with Steve today, not when he was feeling so weak.

But somehow, by the time I made it home, I couldn't hold it in.

Steve lay asleep under the blue blanket I'd draped over the back of the couch earlier. Beside him sat his half-drunk cup of tea, now cold, and some barely nibbled snacks. His appetite was dismal, made worse by his digestive struggles and he'd taken to swallowing handfuls of digestive enzymes with every meal, including snacks. The little bottle of pills lay open next to the barely touched plate of home-made, gluten free biscuits on the side table.

It was difficult watching him literally fading away. He'd lost over 20 kilos in weight since we'd met and now his head, like a fine boned Hollywood actor's, look disproportionately large on his too-svelte frame silhouetted by the blanket.

He woke as I tried to tip toe around in the adjacent kitchen making lunch.

"How are you feeling?" I asked.

"Dreadful," he murmured.

We had our daily discussion about his bowels which had become a significant topic of concern for us both. Opening them usually gave him a short window of relief from the grinding discomfort of the condition. No relief today however, despite several more painful visits to the loo since I'd left earlier that morning.

"Maybe you're a bit dehydrated," I suggested, bringing over a glass of water, warm from the kettle.

He rolled over to prop himself up on a skinny elbow and took a few sips of water. I reflected on how lucky we were that he was still able to move around the house by himself and support his own weight in this way. We had read about others who couldn't – and we were only just coping as it was.

"Any pain?" I asked as I set the glass of water down on his side table.

"Not at the moment," he said, rolling back down and closing his eyes.

I carried on making lunch. We had decided early on in Steven's illness that eating our main meal at lunchtime would be more beneficial for his digestion. It was hard enough for him to digest at all, let alone before bed. Food would sit in his stomach for hours and reflux no matter how many antacids he ingested. Later, we introduced diluted lemon juice and apple cider vinegar drinks, probiotics, psyllium husks and other known dietary aids, as we got better at managing his constitution. He would also take a daily proton pump inhibitor on prescription from his doctor to reduce the acid reflux. Eating his main meal at lunchtime at least gave him a chance to absorb some nutrition.

I got the baking tray out and started to prepare the salmon fillets I'd bought on the way home, plucking out a couple of bones the fish monger had missed. My thoughts turned to Steve's mum who loved to prepare this dish with a dill sauce. Most of the concerns of Steven's family for his health fell around food, his visible and striking weight loss taking almost equal billing with his lack of ability to work. Considering his weight had plummeted so dramatically, coincidentally since he had married me, they naturally regarded me with a high degree of suspicion.

In truth, no one could have been more suspicious of me than I was of myself. I found I was constantly berating myself and wondering what on earth I could have done wrong to transform my healthy, vibrant boyfriend into an incapacitated, ill, frail, and emaciated husband? As soon as we'd tied the knot!

The lack of a firm, believable diagnosis left a vacuum in understanding to be filled, but never between Steve and me. I had a tendency to blame myself when things went wrong, and Steve always encouraged me to go beyond this conclusion and his emotional support despite his ill health was invaluable to me. We were growing together in ways that perhaps our families couldn't see, and they not unsurprisingly took a different view of our union.

In Steve's Mum's eyes it was likely it was the quality of my cooking that was being examined. Regardless of the excellent culinary tuition my mum had imparted to me, Steven was dwindling before my eyes, and I felt like I was failing him and his mum. Later we would meet others with ME/CFS with the same difficulty in keeping weight on. For others it was the opposite problem.

It also wasn't the time for me to quibble about feminist values I held dear about who should be in the kitchen. Steven wasn't even able to stand on the hard flooring in the kitchen for more than a few minutes let alone cook, and he enjoys cooking.

Eating meat caused me some inner conflict, and my vegetarian instincts were starting to emerge back then, so I was routinely asked by our families and even mere acquaintances if Steven was eating enough meat, and did I give him plenty of bread and cake to build him up? Bread and cake were good for weight gain I was reminded! Gluten was a new concept in general conversation, so everyone was concerned about this highly suspicious 'Glutton-free' diet he was on. Increasingly, the contents of my dinner plate at family parties were scrutinised and became a hot topic of discussion, judged to be bird-like and perhaps, even proof of how little I must have been feeding Steven.

In fact, I had the opposite concern. I liked to eat a big main meal, but I knew from experience that my portion sizes were too big for Steve to manage, and so I adapted in order to provide support. Instead of one, big main meal, I served Steven several smaller platefuls across the day. With an effort of will, I selected the smallest fillet of fish for my diminishing partner. Steve was too thin, and I yearned to pile lashings of food on his plate – but I resisted knowing it would only make him worse. I repeated a mantra in my mind, 'less is more, less is more,' and put a smallish spoonful of rice and a few choice veggies on his plate next to the salmon, with a drizzle of pesto and some extra virgin olive oil.

I saved another small salmon fillet in a separate container, and in another, a selection of left-over veggies and rice so Steve could easily reheat them if I happened to be back at work when he felt hungry again. I also set aside the salad dressing in a container and the left-over salad undressed, so it would be palatable later. With barely any energy, Steve had limited capacity to cater for himself, so I tried to make it as easy as possible to give him some independence over his food without exhausting him.

As I busied myself in the kitchen, the conversation I'd had with Dad was still boiling away in my mind, vying for expression, but I knew Steve was in no state to hear it. It's hard to admit but trying to repeatedly put my own needs second was not always easy, but at this time there were even greater forces driving me to speak despite the inappropriate timing.

I was acutely aware of my father's growing intolerance of Steven. We weren't children for goodness' sake, I thought to myself but somehow our fragile situation must have made us appear to him as children again and I knew he wanted to be the best Dad possible to me. I feared Ian was of a mind to intervene, in what way I didn't know.

And so, after we'd finished our meal and I was washing up, I could hold it in no longer. The words slipped out of my mouth before I could stop them.

"Ian wants us to come to Christmas lunch," I found myself saying. "He wants a reply today."

Steve was listening but said nothing.

"He wasn't happy," I said, "he couldn't understand why we hadn't come to Melbourne last month to meet the cousins down from Queensland."

"What did you tell him?" Steve asked.

"That you weren't well enough to travel the three hours to Melbourne. He got cross and said he's heard it all before."

Steve's already pale features were overcome by an ashen pall. He rested his elbows on the table and cradled his head in his hands. This was a definite signal that I had witnessed many times before when Steven's energy reserves were crashing. It was time to cease the conversation, but I couldn't stop. I was so worried my family were on the brink of rejecting him.

"Barry rang Ian again, too," I said and immediately regretted it. Steve let out a groan and retreated to the couch but didn't lie down as his stomach was too full. I could see his whole frame droop.

"What did Doctor Barry say this time?" he said after a long pause. Barry was a retired doctor and old friend of Steven's family.

"He told Dad he doesn't believe in Chronic Fatigue Syndrome."

Silence filled the space between us until the kettle squealed.

"Apparently as far as Barry's concerned, it's nothing a few antidepressants wouldn't fix." I said over the top of the kettle as I struggled to remove my wet washing up gloves to switch it off.

I had always believed in Steve and knew that antidepressants were some of the earliest treatments Steven had tried, but we had agreed along with his GP that they seemed to make things worse. The only dosage he could tolerate was a tiny 10mgs of tricyclics at night to help him sleep.

I was the messenger of this news from Barry, but I suddenly felt like the executioner.

Still wordless, Steve wilted so far down into the sofa, he disappeared from view.

I chastised myself inwardly and went back to washing up. I should have kept it to myself, until a better time. But when would it ever be a better time?

"I can't go to Christmas, you know they don't believe me," came a small voice eventually from the sofa.

This time my shoulders drooped, as my hands swirled like a pair of aimless goldfish in the washing up water. I knew Steve was right.

It wasn't Barry or Ian's fault, I tried to remind myself.

I reflected on the consultation we'd had four years earlier with the psychiatrist who'd confirmed Steven's diagnosis. I always attended Steve's consultations as his attention span was compromised by the brain-fog that came with his condition, and I needed to understand what was happening to him - to us.

The psychiatrist had been a kind and compassionate man, gently explaining that most doctors in Australia gave the diagnosis of ME/CFS little credence. He told us that he was convinced it was a genuine physical illness, he'd seen it in several other patients, some type of autoimmune condition he thought or neurological, and not a psychological problem. He was ahead of his time and his was a lone voice.

I wished I could have talked this over with Ian and Barry.

I wanted to tell them that the psychiatrist had concluded it was clear from his first-hand assessment of Steven, that his problem was consistent with a physical condition that was itself causing the significant mental distress, not the other way around. Unfortunately, he had informed us, there was no diagnostic test that could demonstrate its reality, but he hoped this would come soon.

While this was reassuring advice, it was early on in our experience of ME/CFS. We soon learned this sort of validation was very much not the norm and became increasingly disheartened.

Scraping the carrot peelings off the chopping board into the compost bin, I cringed as I recalled Steve's battle to draw on his income protection claim. Back then, without a recognised diagnostic tool, we were packed off to several eminent specialists for assessment and reassessment. After batteries of negative test results and no diagnostic basket to neatly fit Steven's symptoms into, they decided the problem must be me.

One of the specialists, another psychiatrist, decided it must be that I was failing my husband in the bedroom! This came out of the blue at the end of Steven's interview, without interviewing me, without asking about our sex life or giving Steven a sexual health questionnaire. His conclusion was that at our age we should be making love at least twice a night and I wasn't sufficiently affirming Steven's confidence in his own manliness…Boy if I felt inadequate before this really took the cake!

But hang on! There was an even better explanation. The other specialist, a Professor of Medicine, expressed concern in a letter to our GP that Steven was underweight, and that his skin looked somewhat yellow or jaundiced, even though his liver function tests were normal.

He concluded that I was clearly restricting Steven's meals and replacing them with carrots.

I wish I was joking!

The tragic truth was, those juliennes of shame were triggered once more by Barry's harsh words shared with my father, undermining my already failing confidence as a wife, carer, and daughter and dispiriting us both.

"I think we'll have to consider going to Christmas lunch," I said, "we just have to be organised for every eventuality!"

Attempting to shake off the shame and flailing against the storm that was building in my family I was now talking to myself. Steve had downed another pill and crumpled under the blanket.

Over the next few weeks, I knew I'd be constructing lists, pre-preparing suitable snacks to conceal in my handbag and planning for Steve to rest for days in advance, just so that he would have enough energy in reserve for Christmas day.

I heard myself say as if across no man's land, "it won't matter if it takes you a few days to recover, we'll plan for that too."

At some level, I knew I was deluding myself, but I was torn between loyalty to Steve and loyalty to my father. I pushed away the thought of the PEM Steve would have to endure and was in denial about the other aftermath that would engulf us both.

It would be OK, it would be a military exercise I reasoned to myself, and I would plan it down to the last detail.

I couldn't and wouldn't let Dad and my family down again!

'But what about Steve?' said a little voice in my head.

I ignored it and rang Ian to confirm that we would be attending Christmas lunch.

Three weeks later, to try to normalise family relations, we went to the Christmas family gathering...

With precision planning, careful rest and days of preparation, Steve seemed almost normal in those few hours of snatched time with my family, but the die was cast.

I simply hadn't accounted for the bombs of disbelief that would rain down upon us.

Without any official medical backing and in an effort to try to fit in, we would pay a very high price.

The repercussions of trying to live up to impossible societal expectations that deny anything but vitality in a young person, especially one who had been at the pinnacle of his career, triggered a painful rift between me and my family that is ongoing today.

I learned I could not hope to relieve my family's anxiety about us and was forced to make an unimaginable choice between Steven and my family.

Steve and I remain hopeful of finding acknowledgment and acceptance, especially among those we have held most dear. Their inability to accept our reality has been undeniably difficult on top of everything else – but the flip side is, it has confirmed an unshakeable bond between me and Steve.

My hope is that by sharing this window into my personal experience, it will affirm other people in a caring role and help to bridge the gaps in understanding that can develop with other near and dear in the presence of a loved one dealing with ME/CFS.

People with ME/CFS are highly sensitive to all stimuli in their environment and this could include the person who may be caring for them. It's not personal it is part of the condition, and it can take time to find the right balance between each other. However, it's also not easy so I hope carers find ways to care for themselves too. I'll finish this chapter with a brief reflection on the survival keys I learned as a partner/carer.

- Be kind to yourself, it's not easy and you're doing a great job!
- Learning to ask for help is challenging but essential.
- A supportive GP is invaluable to the person with ME/CFS and to their partner/carer if they have one.
- An ideal counsellor/psychologist for the carer would have an understanding of ME/CFS **and** an understanding of the carer experience. I found this to be rare in the one person so you may need more than one input at different times.
- ME/CFS and carer support groups may have a list of suitable GP's and counsellors.
- A financial counsellor and/or Social Worker is also an invaluable resource. I found Social Workers understood the carer experience better than the psychologists I saw.
- Deep relaxation, meditation and yoga were good practices for me.
- I was able to go out for my own respite once we had some council help in place to cover my time-out from Steven's care.
- If the NDIS is accessible this is an invaluable support.
- Social connection was vital in the absence of family support. Coffees with girlfriends kept me going.
- I discovered a love of art and drawing and found inexpensive art classes through the local community center that gave me friendships as well as a wonderful hobby.
- As a carer it is almost inevitable you will feel every emotion along with anger at times and this is completely normal. I certainly did and had times when I failed to reign it in and caused hurt to people that I loved. It's best to work through it with a counsellor/ psychologist rather than unleashing it on anyone near and dear, especially your ill loved one.
- You may feel trapped or burnt out as a carer or in a situation you didn't expect to find yourself in. I had times like this and found it the hardest emotional experience to cope with. This could occur if your partner, your parent, or even your child has ME/CFS. A friend of ours nursed her daughter-in-law. It's also completely understandable and normal to feel overwhelmed at times. Be proactive, seek help and find someone or someway that works for you, to help you to cope with this. You **can** come through it and find the answers you need.
- Slowly Steve and I learned to let go of long cherished expectations. We began to enjoy the life we did have even if it was not the life we expected.
- Now we are embracing life again and the strange journey it has taken us on!

CARER SURVIVAL KEYS

Chapter 10

MULTISYSTEM MALFUNCTION - THE EVIDENCE

PART 1 MITOCHONDRIAL DYSFUNCTION AND THE HIBERNATION SWITCH

"Which came first the chicken or the egg."

PLUTARCH

It is possible that the recent discovery of neuro-inflammation in the brain on PET scans we looked at in Chapter 5 is responsible for all the various malfunctioning systems that had been discovered by ME/CFS researchers prior to this. It is also possible it could be the other way around. For example, an over-reacting immune system may have led to the release of inflammatory cytokines (I will explain shortly) which in themselves cause symptoms. Some of these cytokines may also be the cause of the noted neuro-inflammation.

Of course, both may be occurring simultaneously as well as involving other combinations of bodily systems. One thing we keep learning in medical science is that everything is connected, nonetheless, looking at specific systems in turn can also help us understand the whole, if we stay open to the possibilities.

So, to make the whole more visible, over the next three chapters we will look at specific research demonstrating biomedical dysfunction as it relates to various body systems affected by or affecting ME/CFS.

To make the relevance of this research clearer, each chapter will begin with the symptoms (in italics) a person with ME/CFS may have, aligning them with the Canadian Diagnostic Clinical Criteria - CDCC (See Appendix 1) and the body system(s) being discussed.

We'll begin by exploring the ground-breaking discoveries surrounding mitochondrial energy production, then in Chapters 11 and 12, review research covering the Neuroendocrine system, the Autonomic Nervous System and Immune Systems.

If research is not your thing then by all means, skip ahead any time you wish. Otherwise, here we go.

Energy Production

Our bodies need energy to function, even while we are asleep. Our brain requires more energy than any other organ. We produce energy via two main biochemical pathways:

By converting food slowly with oxygen (**aerobic metabolism**) into energy.

By converting food quickly without oxygen (**anaerobic metabolism**) into energy.

This energy production occurs within the cells of the body, aerobic within the many mitochondria ('energy batteries') within each cell; anaerobic still within the cell but not within the mitochondria. Aerobic energy production takes many chemical steps to achieve but produces 19 times more energy per glucose molecule than anaerobic energy production. When we rest or exercise within our capacities, aerobic pathways are at play. While oxygen and food are available, these aerobic chemical pathways can be used for long periods of time as they do not produce harmful waste products, like lactic acid (lactate), that, by contrast, is produced during the faster, more readily available anaerobic energy production.[1,2]

In truth we can be flipping between both methods of energy production as a day unfolds. It's when we exercise that things become more obvious.

For example, a healthy person strolling easily, walking well within their capabilities, will use aerobic metabolism to fuel this activity until they suddenly need to sprint to catch a train and briefly switch to fast-twitch muscle fibers that use anaerobic metabolism for fuel.

This is especially notable in the Olympics. An athlete-sprinter competing in the 100-metre dash will quickly reach what's called the 'anaerobic threshold' where they move from the more sustainable aerobic to the more rapid, but time limited anaerobic energy production. By comparison, marathon runners try to stay just underneath this threshold, timing their brief final burst to be as short as possible. If they misjudge this, as you may have seen on TV, the lactate build-up in the blood stream from anerobic metabolism will literally slow them to a halt or even cripple them, causing them to collapse completely as their muscles seize up.

An interesting factoid is that humans outperform every other mammal on this planet in endurance running, due to the marvelous efficient aerobic energy production that occurs within our mitochondria.

But how is this relevant to ME/CFS? Let's check out some symptoms.

CDCC Appendix 1

1. **(a) Pathological fatigue** *A significant degree of new onset, unexplained, persistent or recurrent physical and/or mental fatigue that substantially reduces activity levels and which is not the result of ongoing exertion and not relieved by rest.*

   (b) Post-exertional malaise *Mild exertion or even normal activities followed by malaise: the loss of physical and mental stamina and/or worsening of other symptoms. Both onset and recovery can be delayed, taking more than 24 hours.*

   (c) Stress *of any kind can aggravate symptoms.*

2. **Sleep problems** *Sleep is un-refreshing: disturbed quantity - daytime hypersomnia or night-time insomnia and/or disturbed rhythm – day/night reversal. Rarely is there no sleep problem.*

3. **Pain** *Pain is widespread, migratory or localized: Myalgia; arthralgia (without signs of inflammation); and/or headache - a new type, pattern or severity. Rarely is there no pain.*

4. **Neurological/Cognitive Manifestations** *(Two Neurocognitive symptoms) Impaired concentration, short term memory or word retrieval; hypersensitivity to light, noise or emotional overload; confusion; disorientation; slowness of thought; muscle weakness; ataxia.*

Mitochondrial Dysfunction

We now know that people with ME/CFS have a malfunction in **aerobic metabolism within the mitochondria**. As mentioned above, mitochondria are tiny oblong shaped organelles within most of the cells of the body. A human cell can house anywhere from two to 2500 mitochondria within it and this number can change depending on your fitness. As you'd expect they are most plentiful in muscle cells and cells of the heart where energy needs to be readily available. The evidence now suggests that problems generating and using the main energy molecule, adenosine triphosphate (ATP), within the mitochondria may be a fundamental driver of ME/CFS. The ATP production pathway problem is more pronounced in severe ME/CFS than in people with more moderate versions.

The significance of this mitochondrial problem in ME/CFS has been confirmed by cardiopulmonary exercise testing (CPET).[3] As I've explained above, the anaerobic system is only designed for fast, short-term use and produces lactic acid (lactate).

In people with ME/CFS, CPET research confirms that the aerobic metabolism, while not fully broken, is incapacitated and shorter lived than normal. Therefore, if people with ME/CFS participate in enforced maximal exercise, like cycling as fast as they can, their anaerobic threshold is crossed very early on. Then having to rely upon anaerobic energy production, they readily build up lactate levels in their bloodstream. This is especially obvious if there is a repeated exercise session 24-hours after the initial exercise session.

Lactic acid can cause inflammation leading to muscle pain and can harm the body in other ways. By comparison, 'well but sedentary people,' or people affected by a number of other chronic illnesses, when asked to exercise to their maximal ability on 2 consecutive days, their energy test results do not change significantly from one day to the next. They may not use oxygen as efficiently as healthy, physically fit people, but their energy efficiency remains the same on repeated testing.[4]

By contrast, in ME/CFS, the ability to generate energy deteriorates on a repeated test the second day. Not surprisingly then, the people with ME/CFS tested in this way ended up unwell for weeks with Post-exertional malaise (PEM) following this form of testing, while the sedentary people felt healthier and reduced their levels of lactate after their second test 24 hours later![5]

Let's be clear, repeated exercise improves lactic acid disposal in healthy people and other conditions but not in ME/CFS. You would therefore expect the muscles to be inflamed by this excess lactate and they are. A review paper in 2017 confirmed the findings of low-grade inflammation in the muscles of people with ME/CFS. The paper concluded, "The presence of chronic oxidative and nitrosative stress, low-grade inflammation and impaired heat shock protein production (reducing the capacity for the muscle to repair itself) may well explain the objective findings of increased muscle fatigue, impaired contractility and multiple dimensions of exercise intolerance in many patients with ME/CFS."[6]

Moreover, compared with patients moderately affected with ME/CFS, **severely** affected patients not only have problems generating energy using oxygen via the aerobic pathway but also had a poorly functioning anaerobic (known as glycolytic) pathway as well.[7] Damage to more than one energy generation system (ie aerobic and anaerobic) may account for why severely affected patients are often so limited in what they can do each day.

In addition to this, as we will discover in Chapter 12, the release of proinflammatory chemicals from immune cells known as cytokines has also been a confirmed contributor to exercise intolerance and post exertional malaise (PEM).

Research also indicates that if PEM occurs, subsequent exercise capacity will be even more limited until the PEM resolves. Hence, just as healthy people with a nasty flu-like illness are unwise to try to push on with previous exercise routines until they recover, so too when PEM occurs in people with ME/CFS, even a limited routine may need to be reduced or ceased until the PEM passes.

Also, people with ME/CFS may unwittingly exert themselves beyond their aerobic threshold at such low levels of activity so as not to be considered exercising at all and wonder why they have crashed.

Stopping all physical activity is not the answer either. This is crucial as respected ME/CFS researcher Nancy Klimas puts it, "You must find a way to exercise safely, because if you do not exercise you will get worse."[8,9] We'll look at this issue more closely in Chapter 13, but suffice to say for now, that these research findings have blown up the speculations of those physicians and scientists who suggested that these exertional limitations were due to physical deconditioning or an irrational fear of activity. In the companion book we will look at how to safely navigate this very real limitation in some detail (*ME/CFS – A Path back to Life - the Art of Micro-Rehab*).

Lessons from the Dauer - Hypometabolic 'Hibernation' Response?

The new science of metabolomics looks at metabolites, which are very small chemicals that are produced **inside** body cells. This includes the biochemical reactions involved within the mitochondria that produce the energy as we've just been exploring. Much like the characteristic algorithm patterns of cytokines (messengers **between** body cells) there appears to be similar characteristic patterns of metabolites related to specific illnesses.[10]

One impressive study in this field of research, found very definite patterns of metabolites in people with ME/CFS that were consistent with a hypometabolic state, that is, a low-energy (or could it be hibernation?) state.

The metabolic signatures were different between men and women with ME/CFS, but there was an overlap of nine common metabolites that were shared by both sexes. The presence of these particular patterns predicted, with about **90%** accuracy, whether the person had ME/CFS or was healthy! Once again, like the cytokine algorithms we'll explore in Chapter 12, it also found it could predict which cases of ME/CFS were the most severe. Much more research is needed to clarify these findings, but in time this knowledge may lead to a simplified blood test for ME/CFS.[11] Beyond this it raises some fascinating questions.

Is it possible that humans still have a primitive hibernation brain 'switch,' like other creatures such as bears? The well-researched worm known as the Dauer (picture a worm in an apple as these worms are Dauer worms) exhibits this trait. These worms can literally put their bodies into a stand-by hibernation type state where energy is conserved when conditions are poor (e.g. lack of food, cool temperatures etc.) or if they feel threatened in other ways. If so, this may be a hidden trait in humans. It could well be that we also have a brainstem survival epigenetic switching mechanism that activates under certain conditions and may present as very severe ME/CFS. People with a predisposition to developing ME/CFS may be vulnerable to this ancient low-energy pathway switch being turned on in response to **serious threats**, be they infectious, chemical, traumatic (physical or psychological) or any combination of these.[12]

Recall the Dubbo Study (Ch 6) which found the **severity of the illness** experienced, regardless of the cause, was the key predictor of whether an individual would go on to develop ME/CFS.[13] This would correlate with an epigenetic hibernation switch.

Importantly, an epigenetic switch can be switched off or on. Bears and worms can come out of hibernation fit and well. Intriguingly, this may explain why in a few people with ME/CFS to whom I taught specific mind-body techniques, there was an apparent sudden improvement only to revert backwards just as quickly, literally like the flick of a switch.

On the other hand, I have witnessed when people adopted a persistent and patient (as neuroplasticity requires for change) holistic approach to their restoration it was more likely to be steadier and to hold into the future as their survival imperative became less concerning. In this circumstance, as adequate supports were put in place and hope from feeling improvement with Micro-Rehab was experienced, the hibernation switch was slowly but surely switched off and life returned. (We'll explore this further in *ME/CFS – A Path Back to Life*).

Carbohydrate Metabolism Weakness?

Other metabolomic researchers are finding people with ME/CFS are unable to efficiently convert carbohydrate foods (think white foods such as sugar, rice, bread, spuds, bananas etc.) into energy due to a possible autoimmune response. The enzyme pyruvate dehydrogenase (PDH) is very important in the biochemical reactions within the mitochondria responsible for converting glucose and oxygen into energy. They postulate that a trigger, like an infection, causes the body's immune system to see the PDH enzyme as a foreign invader to be attacked. A lack of PDH, and maybe other enzymes as well, could be responsible for the poor aerobic metabolism in the mitochondria we discussed previously and thus would explain the quickly fatiguing and painful muscles in ME/CFS, that can occur with minimal over-exertion.[14]

Dr Chris Armstrong a metabolomic researcher at Melbourne University when interviewed by New Scientist said, "Together, these metabolic approaches are suggesting that ME/CFS has a chemical cause." He continued, "It's definitely a physiological effect that we're observing, and not psychosomatic, and I'll put my head on the block on that."[15]

In Chapter 14, Epigenetic switches, we will explore how it would be possible, even with a predisposing genetic code, *to alter genetic expression* and potentially recover from ME/CFS.

Chapter 10
Key Points

✓ Once postulated to be a purely hysterical psychological disorder, this is now debunked. Research using the latest technology has and continues to confirm we are dealing with a distinctive illness affecting multiple body systems.

✓ Neuro-endocrine, autonomic nervous system dysfunction and energy production dysfunction relating to the aerobic metabolism within mitochondria are all evidence of a multisystem disease.

✓ Mitochondria are tiny organelles within cells that play a critical role in energy production.

✓ People with severe ME/CFS also have a malfunctioning anaerobic (glycolytic) energy producing pathway as well as an aerobic malfunction.

✓ The study of Metabolomics has posed the intriguing hypothesis of an ancient energy-conserving hibernation 'switch' being triggered which may yet explain much about ME/CFS. This switch may occur in the brainstem.

MULTISYSTEM MALFUNCTION – THE EVIDENCE

PART 2 NEURO-ENDOCRINE AND AUTONOMIC NERVOUS SYSTEM

Appendix 1 CCDC 5B Neuroendocrine *Low body temperature; cold extremities; sweating; intolerance to heat or cold; reduced tolerance for stress; other symptoms worsen with stress; weight change; abnormal appetite (Up or Down).*

One or more of the following neuroendocrine abnormalities has been found in studies of patients with ME/CFS. Some of the research facts listed are quite technical so feel free to skip ahead if you like. I include them here for the scientists amongst you.

- Reduced function of the Hypothalamic Pituitary Adrenal (HPA) axis is often referred to as Adrenal Exhaustion. This can follow on from a period of overdrive with feelings of high stress/anxiety secondary to activation of the sympathetic (fight/flight) nervous system and can lead to measurable increased levels of cortisol in saliva, urine and blood, released from the Adrenal gland. As this situation becomes chronic and exhaustion sets in, lower levels of cortisol become apparent and there is less diurnal variation, suggesting less flexibility to respond to daily life appropriately.

Note: The HPA axis extends its influence beyond the adrenal glands to the thyroid and gonad (sex hormone) function as well.[1-3]

- Raised levels of neuropeptide Y (released in the brain and sympathetic nervous system following stress) is possibly linked to the dysfunction of the HPA axis. Neuropeptide Y levels in plasma have been correlated with symptom severity.[4]

- Blunted Cortisol response to ACTH (a pituitary hormone) injection despite normal baseline levels.[5] This test is mostly done by endocrinologists to assess the function of the HPA axis.

- Low IGF1 (Insulin Growth Factor also called somatomedin) levels and an exaggerated growth hormone response to pyridostigmine.[6] Another specialist pathology test.

- Increased prolactin (a pituitary hormone with a role in lactation) response to buspirone.[7]

- A disturbance of fluid metabolism as evidenced by low baseline levels of arginine vasopressin, which can influence blood pressure.[8]

- Relatively lower levels of aldosterone (an adrenal hormone) in patients compared with controls can contribute to low blood pressure and fatigue.[9] The presence of increased Heart Rate and reduced Heart Rate Variability in ME/CFS during sleep coupled with higher norepinephrine (also known as noradrenaline, an adrenal hormone and neurotransmitter in the sympathetic nervous system) levels and lower plasma aldosterone suggest a state of sympathetic autonomic nervous system predominance. This means the fight and flight response is overactive making coping with stress very difficult. This was evident in my own experience (see my story in Chapter 4).

Autonomic Nervous System Dysfunction (Dysautonomia)

Appendix 1 CCDC 5A Autonomic

Orthostatic intolerance: neurally mediated hypotension (NMH) i.e. low blood pressure can be a delayed onset occurring after up to 10 minutes of standing; postural orthostatic tachycardia (POTS); light headedness; extreme pallor; palpitations; exertional dyspnea (shortness of breath); urinary frequency; irritable bowel syndrome (IBS); nausea.

We touched upon some of the wide-ranging roles the Autonomic Nervous System (ANS) plays in our bodies when we looked at the brainstem in Chapter 5. It largely does this via the far travelling vagus nerve, the longest nerve of the ANS (vagus derives from the latin meaning wandering or rambling). It arises from the brainstem carrying messages in its many branches via the Sympathetic Nervous System ('Flight/fight or freeze') and the Parasympathetic Nervous System ('Rest and digest') to and from the rest of the body. This includes heart, lungs, blood vessels, stomach and intestines (small and large) and all the other organs in the abdomen (kidneys, adrenals, pancreas, liver, spleen etc.). Hence, dysautonomia can have widespread negative effects. As the symptoms above suggest, this can range from blood pressure to breathlessness to irritable bowel or bladder to poor digestion.

Most people with ME/CFS have low blood pressure (BP) as I did; and this is worse whilst standing. One of my patients would faint several times a day at work due to low blood pressure. This said, blood pressure can fluctuate widely with some people noting a sharp rise in their BP on lying down. So, your doctor may suggest a 5-day home heart rate and BP measuring device to assess this.

Chronotropic Intolerance (CI)

Since the CCDC was established in 2003, there has been the discovery of another way in which dysautonomia affects the heart. It has been found that many people with ME/CFS have chronotropic intolerance (CI).

Analysis has revealed that smaller or reduced increases in heart rate during cardiopulmonary exercise testing (CPET) are consistently observed in ME/CFS. This blunted/sluggish rise in heart rate is called chronotropic intolerance (CI). CI reflects an inability to appropriately increase cardiac output because of smaller than expected increases in heart rate.[10]

When we exercise, more oxygen is required to be pumped around the body in our bloodstream so that energy can be produced in our muscles to meet the increased need.

For this to happen, Cardiac Output (CO) needs to rise. [CO=HR x Stroke Volume (SV)]. SV is the amount of blood pumped out by the heart with each beat. So, if your heart rate is not increasing as it should, then CO will not increase in proportion to the need and these muscles will not receive the oxygen they will be 'screaming for.' Hence, they will have to rapidly revert to anaerobic sources of energy leading to a quick build-up of lactic acid (lactate).[11] [I describe what it was like for me to experience Chronotropic Intolerance (CI) in Chapter 15.

A review paper published in 2019 collated all ME/CFS CPET research documenting 2,270 people with ME/CFS and comparing them to 594 controls. They found on CPET an average rise of **11.2 heart beats per minute less** in the people with ME/CFS. This CI coincided with a **92% lower performance** than in controls.[12] This is another significant autonomic nervous system dysfunction that could explain some of the serious limitations the illness imposes.

Chapter 11
Key Points

✓ Neuroendocrine abnormalities involving the HPA axis have long been known to be a contributor to fatigue states. In ME/CFS this is just one of many neuroendocrine factors implicated.

✓ Dysautonomia contributes to blood pressure problems, low blood pressure most commonly. The recent discovery of Chronotropic Intolerance (CI), where the heart is sluggish off the mark in response to exercise, may allow new treatment strategies to be investigated, starting with specific brief exercise interventions.

Chapter 12

MULTISYSTEM MALFUNCTION - THE EVIDENCE

PART 3 IMMUNE SYSTEM

Immune Dysfunction

Appendix 1 CCDC 5 (c) Immune *Recurrent flu-like symptoms; sore throats; tender lymph nodes; fevers; new sensitivities to food, medicines, odors or chemicals.*

Our immune system is a finely tuned and highly intelligent defense force. It keeps a record of every foreign invader (antigen) it encounters in our lifetime so that if that antigen is encountered again, it is quickly recognized and eliminated. In this way it protects us (it is how immunizations work). However, it can sometimes get it wrong. If it incorrectly sees a part of our-self as foreign and/or over-reacts to the detected threat, acute allergic reactions or chronic autoimmune conditions can result. Many scientists believe that ultimately ME/CFS will be classified as an autoimmune disease.[1]

Our white blood cells (leukocytes) are our bodies major Defense Force and in the last decade have been the subject of extensive research as to their relationship to ME/CFS. You see, as a part of the elimination process involving an antigen invader, certain leukocytes will sometimes be called upon to release chemicals that help to destroy the invader. Some of these chemicals, known as cytokines, are used to communicate within the immune system and some can cause inflammation and flu-like symptoms.

The first recognized cytokine was a chemical known as interferon. Interferon has now been produced in different forms to treat some cancers and chronic viral infections such as hepatitis C. When interferon is injected as a treatment for cancer or viruses, its side-effects are flu-like, much like PEM, confirming a likely role of cytokines in the production of the symptoms manifesting in ME/CFS.

Is Post-exertional Malaise (PEM) 'Real?'

A decade-long exploration into cytokine release in ME/CFS, eventually led to a review of 23 studies that looked at whether post-exertional malaise (PEM) had a corresponding biological basis. In other words, do people affected by ME/CFS truly respond differently to exercise and if so, can this be measured physically/chemically? This review compared the bodily responses to exercise testing in healthy sedentary people and people with ME/CFS. We looked at this in Chapter 10 with regards to aerobic energy production and lactic acid build up. This review was looking more at cytokines and immune responses after maximal exercise. What did they find?

They consistently found significant differences in the way the immune system responded in the people affected by ME/CFS when compared with healthy sedentary people.[2] People with ME/CFS who experienced a significant symptom flare post-exercise showed increased inflammatory cytokines in blood samples taken eight hours later.[3] These differences combined with the lactic acid build up due to CI (see Chapter 11) could explain some of the flu-like symptoms of PEM that occur in response to overexertion in people with ME/CFS.

The Turning Point - SEID is born

In 2015 the independent and respected non-profit Institute of Medicine in the United States (now known as the National Academy of Medicine), reviewed the ME/CFS research literature and published a report that concluded there was *"sufficient evidence to support the finding of immune dysfunction in ME/CFS."*[4-7] This was the origin of the proposal to rename ME/CFS as Systemic Exertional Intolerance Disease (SEID).

While not all patients exhibit every one of these abnormal immune system dysfunctions in response to over-exertion, most exhibit some. In the minds of researchers at least, if one was to select a **turning point** where ME/CFS became established as a biomedical **disease rather than a syndrome** of disordered physical and psychological symptoms/ signs, this would be it.

In the US it is accepted by insurance companies that ME/CFS can be diagnosed by two successive exercise tolerance tests done over two consecutive days. If the maximal exercise tolerance test is markedly failed on the second day, it is accepted proof of the existence of ME/ CFS by the medical insurers. However, pushing people like this can leave them sick for many days or weeks or more with PEM. If possible, it's better, under supervision, to use the standardized 10-minute NASA Lean test presented in Chapter 3, although as we've mentioned a simple diagnostic blood test may not be far away.

Immune Dysfunction – Specific Examples

As alluded to above, the abnormal release of cytokines can be responsible for ill-health. Cytokines are small proteins that assist communication between immune cells and influence their behavior. It has been found that cytokine networks, essential in balancing immune function in us all, form a different geometric arrangement in people affected by ME/ CFS than in healthy people. This pattern is consistent with a latent (dormant) viral infection (e.g. like a Herpes 'cold sore' virus that lays dormant until you are fatigued and feeling run down.).[8]

There is also a clear correlation with disease severity linked to the important Natural Killer (NK) leucocyte, which functions poorly in people with ME/CFS. NK cells are best known, as the name suggests, for their role in killing cells infected by viruses as well as in the detection and destruction of tumor cells in the early stages of cancer. In people affected by ME/CFS, there is a correlation between Natural Killer cell function and the degree of severity of the condition. The lower the level of NK functioning, the more severe the illness and the more disturbed is cognitive function.[9-11]

Researchers have also correlated daily fatigue severity with inflammation in a study of adipokine leptin (a cytokine) in women with ME/CFS. This correlation with fatigue levels and inflammation was not seen in healthy women. Just by analyzing this leptin's behavior alone, a computer learning algorithm differentiated high from low fatigue days in the ME/CFS group with 78.3% accuracy![12,13] These correlations help to explain the **physical chemical reasons** why people with ME/CFS are feeling unwell.

A Simple Diagnostic Blood Test?

Now that ME/CFS is accepted as a biomedical disease, the race is on amongst ME/CFS researchers to come up with an affordable diagnostic blood test. For example, as I mentioned in Chapter 3, researchers at Griffith University in Australia have discovered a characteristic defective calcium ion receptor on the surface of the Natural Killer immune cell (known as TRPM3) in people with ME/CFS. This faulty receptor impairs the movement of calcium from outside the cell to inside the cell which is likely to have global ill-effects throughout the body.[14] Correlations between cytokine profiles and illness severity as presented above also provide promise for an affordable blood test.[15,16] As discussed in Chapter 10, metabolite profiles may also serve this purpose. These approaches may not only help to diagnose ME/CFS but could also grade its severity.

Chapter 12
Key Points

✓ In 2015 the independent and respected non-profit Institute of Medicine in the United States (now known as the National Academy of Medicine), reviewed the ME/CFS research literature and published a report that concluded there was *"sufficient evidence to support the finding of immune dysfunction in ME/CFS."* This was the origin of the proposal to rename ME/CFS as Systemic Exertional Intolerance Disease (SEID)

✓ Since 2015 many more research studies confirm multiple immune system abnormalities in people with ME/CFS. Cytokine profiles can predict the severity of the illness, as can the level of Natural Killer Cell dysfunction. This research may soon lead to a simple diagnostic blood test, both to diagnose and to confirm the severity of ME/CFS.

✓ Delineating the subtypes of ME/CFS may help hone treatment strategies in future as increasing research brings increased understanding.

✓ It is, however, possible to safely improve prognosis by putting into practice the holistic rehabilitation principles I will share in *A Path Back to Life – The Art of Micro-Rehab.*

✓ Below is a summary table of key research findings from Chapters 5 to 12.

1. Genetic susceptibility confirmed by twin studies. In Chapter 14, Epigenetic Switches, we will explore how it could be possible, even with a predisposing genetic code, *to alter genetic expression* and recover or significantly improve a disease including, ME/CFS.

2. Multi-system dysfunction: e.g. Immune (SEID) - particular cytokine patterns & response to overexertion; Autonomic Nervous System - POTS, NMH, CI and Endocrine - HPA Axis Overdrive -Adrenal exhaustion with low DHEA etc.

3. Mitochondrial dysfunction as one would expect in a fatiguing neurological disorder, confirmed by metabolomic studies along with impaired heat shock protein production (diminishing muscle repair capacity).

4. Distinctive abnormalities in immune function proportional to disease severity, with the release of cytokines causing flu-like symptoms. The first recognized cytokine was interferon. Interferon has now been produced in different forms to treat some cancers and chronic viral infections such as hepatitis C. When interferon is injected as a treatment for cancer or viruses, its side-effects are PEM/flu-like, confirming a likely link with cytokines in the production of the symptoms manifesting in ME/CFS.

5. Metabolomic research confirms hypometabolic (Hibernation-like) metabolism with measurements of specific metabolite levels proportional to disease severity.

6. Distinctive neurological abnormalities in the brain as evidenced by MRI and fMRI scans indicating:

    a. an increase in white matter in the pre-frontal cortex.
    b. Positron Emission Tomography (PET) studies detecting widespread brain inflammation with consistent involvement of the midbrain (located in the brainstem and critical for autonomic nervous system function).
    c. Once again, the level of inflammation and white matter increase was proportional to disease severity.

Table 1 Evidence for Biological Basis for ME/CFS Summary Table

Before we move closer to my epigenetic turn around, to avoid a major pitfall we need to explore the widely misunderstood topic of exercise as rehabilitation, for in people with ME/CFS it has the power to hurt or to heal.

Chapter 13

BEYOND GET
(GRADED EXERCISE THERAPY)

"You must find a way to exercise safely.
If you do not exercise you will get worse."

DR NANCY KLIMAS, LEADING ME/CFS RESEARCHER AND CLINICIAN AT
INIM (INSTITUTE FOR NEURO-IMMUNE MEDICINE, NOVA SOUTHEASTERN
UNIVERSITY IN FLORIDA)[1]

In my own journey and those I've advised with ME/CFS, finding a way to increase movement appropriately and safely was the tricky key to returning to a healthier state. With post exertional malaise (PEM) lurking it can be potentially fraught. Hence, there are legitimate reasons, as I will explain, why the topic of exercise has been a hot one in ME/CFS circles. It desperately needs clarification for as you will see, it can literally make or break the entire future of someone with this disease.

In the previous three chapters I've presented evidence largely conducted since 2010. This evidence confirms the fact that post exertional malaise (PEM) is a real biomedical reality; most likely related to abnormalities in immune cell release of pro-inflammatory cytokines, aerobic metabolism and autonomic nervous system dysfunction.[2-7]

Prior to 2010, before we were aware of these biomedical abnormalities, ME/CFS was considered and treated by many as a psychiatric problem with secondary physical deconditioning. This physical deconditioning with loss of muscle and bone, rather than being seen as a secondary issue, albeit an important one, was targeted as a way of treating the **whole** problem.

One method of treatment devised by clinicians and researchers was called Graded Exercise Therapy (GET). It involved rigid incremental increases in aerobic exercise (e.g. walking, cycling, swimming) and had very mixed results, some of which I'll share shortly.

Recently GET was officially, and I believe rightly, removed as a recommended treatment option for ME/CFS by the National Institute for Health and Care Excellence (NICE) in the UK.[8]

Unfortunately, while GET has become a dirty word it has tainted all references to the wider topic of exercise. For many in ME/CFS circles this was originally driven by the need to affirm the reality of their very real disease. Now the affirmation fight has been won, since 2015 in fact (I'll explain shortly). However, this battle for recognition has been so traumatic, that it has left behind a **subconscious** trace or mantra, if you like, in the minds of many advocate groups for people with ME/CFS which goes something like this:

"Like lemon juice always curdles milk, **any** exercise always worsens ME/CFS."

Right for lemon juice, wrong for 'any exercise'.

In fact, research and clinical experience point to subtler answers. These answers tell us that tainting ALL approaches to introducing appropriate physical movement in ME/CFS in a negative way is, as Spock (as in Star Trek) would say, "illogical." It is also very dangerous, I'll tell you why in a moment. So where has this anti-all-exercise advice arisen?

To GET or not to GET?

As I've alluded to above, Graded Exercise Therapy (GET) has been the most researched approach to introducing exercise to people with ME/CFS. Often GET involved rigid protocols with regular increases in exercise activity, regardless of how the person with ME/CFS felt.

This focused regime may have been good for researchers wanting to standardize an 'exercise treatment,' but was not good for many people with ME/CFS.

In hindsight and armed with the latest research we can see it was a foolish prescription. Not surprisingly member surveys by ME/CFS societies found up to 60% of participants prescribed GET say they were made worse not better by this prescription.[9-11]

The SEID (Systemic Exertional Intolerance Disease) 2015 Pronouncement

As discussed in Chapter 12, in 2015 the respected non-profit and independent Institute of Medicine, now named the National Academy of Medicine, proposed Systemic Exertional Intolerance Disease (SEID) as an alternate name for ME/CFS. This was a public recognition, on the back of extensive reviews of the biomedical research, that the physiology and biochemistry of people with ME/CFS responded differently to exertion than that of healthy people. Not only this, but the level of severity of their symptoms was proportional to the level of inflammatory cytokines detected in blood tests.[12-14]

If GET researchers pre-2010 had known this, it would have explained to them why the timetable of rigid increases in exercise activity led to a deterioration in the health of participants with ME/CFS that was not 'merely psychosomatic.' Nonetheless, the application of GET by researchers varied and there were some useful lessons to learn here, so let's take a look at two examples.

GET Research - a Tale of Two Approaches

To contrast the differences in how GET was introduced by different researchers let's compare two studies, both conducted around the same era (2004/5) a decade prior to the SEID pronouncement. (Note: This correlates with the time that I was introduced to GET by Dr Lewis, see Chapter 15).

University of Georgia GET Study

Firstly, a study by Christopher Black and Kevin McCully from the University of Georgia in the US involved an enforced 28% increase in daily activity for both a group of healthy sedentary people (the control group) and people with ME/CFS. As we would expect with todays' knowledge, all participants with ME/CFS crashed within 4 to 10 days of commencement, resulting in exercise intolerance and reduced total activity.[15] By contrast, sedentary controls could handle this daily increase and improved their fitness. This study helped to confirm the fact, later proven, that people with ME/CFS do respond differently than healthy people when they exercise.[16]

University of WA GET Study

Compare this with another GET trial conducted by Karen Wallman and colleagues in Perth, Australia and reported in The Medical Journal of Australia in 2004.[17] In this 12-week randomized controlled trial, study participants with ME/CFS were randomly assigned to one of two groups.

1. A submaximal symptom-contingent (effectively paced) graded exercise program.

Or

2. A relaxation/flexibility session twice daily.

All were provided support for remaining as active as possible within the limits imposed by ME/CFS.

The symptom-contingent graded **exercise** group chose either walking, cycling or swimming **second daily**. Increases in exercise were advised *ONLY when people affected by ME/CFS felt they were coping with their current activity levels.* This was determined by average scores on a rating of perception of effort (RPE) scale (see Appendix 3) and heart rate monitoring. Unlike the previous study above by Black and McCully, exercise sessions were **second daily, submaximal and carefully self-monitored.**

As I found with my own recovery program (see Chapter 15) regular 2nd daily sub-maximal aerobic exercise was the aim. In Wallman's study going no further than 75% of full heart capacity was the level recommended and defined as 'sub-maximal'. Other researchers now suggest 60 to 65%. As most people with ME/CFS are not training to be athletes, but rather using this increase in movement as a medicine to recover condition and stamina, I recommend building up slowly to 60% of heart rate capacity, as I did in my own rehab. This care is particularly important as Chronotropic Intolerance (CI – sluggish rise in HR in response to exertion) appears to be a key factor in triggering PEM.

In *A Path Back to Life*, I describe this process as 'Micro-Rehab' and devote several chapters describing how to safely introduce this life-restoring movement.

Professional athletes and people who find this too easy a target, might like to test themselves further. But I would not be recommending anyone diagnosed with ME/CFS go beyond the 70% heart rate, unless strictly supervised in an exercise laboratory.

The Perth research team, most importantly, and in contrast to rigid graded exercise approaches (like Black and Mc Cully's protocol), directed people to stop, not push through, if they experienced symptoms indicating a potential PEM relapse. If symptoms became worse, they could either cancel the session or reduce their level of activity to what they felt able to manage. The twelve-week program involved a fortnightly phone check-in by the same exercise physiologist who performed the initial assessment, along with a face to face follow up a month later, where the final assessments were tallied.

The results? Of the 32 people with ME/CFS who were enrolled in the active program, none felt that the paced rehab made them worse, and 91% of the participants rated themselves as 'better' in respect to their overall health. This was reflected in measurable statistically significant improvements in work capacity, blood pressure readings, cognitive function, mood and stamina. In contrast, the control group of 29 people with ME/CFS, who instead of paced rehab participated in flexibility stretching sessions twice daily, demonstrated none of these improvements at the 12-week follow-up.[18]

'Any exercise' is not the enemy. The approach taken to its introduction is the key. The Perth researchers' protocol would be appropriate for milder and moderate cases of ME/CFS. As you'll see in *A Path Back to Life – The Art of Micro-Rehab*, a much subtler approach may be needed to begin with. This Micro-Rehab approach caters for and can then be applied to the whole spectrum of severity, even the severely deconditioned and/or bedbound/housebound people.

UK PACE Trial Research Confuddles

Despite small trials that have shown promise for both GET (like Wallman's) and Cognitive Behavioral Therapy (CBT) and were initially reported favorably by Cochrane reviews (the gold standard in determining clinical research),[19,20] a definitive answer was still needed. The trouble was, many of these GET trials were neither large enough nor alike-enough in their methodology and they were often appropriately criticized as having inadequately designed protocols. In addition, as mentioned above, surveys of people with ME/CFS reported GET to be harmful in 60% of people.[21-23] In response to all of this, a large study was proposed to hopefully settle the issue once and for all.

The PACE Study

The UK Medical Research Council PACE trial was published in the prestigious Lancet Medical Journal in 2011. This £5 million study was funded by the UK government and was supported by Action for ME, the largest ME/CFS patient advocate group in the UK. The trial was an attempt by the UK government to firmly establish the treatment protocols for people with ME/CFS. The hope was that this would allow those with ME/CFS to qualify for an NHS (National Health Service) approved program and be a win win for all.

The study involved 641 people with ME/CFS and was designed to 'definitively' answer the question about whether exercise in the form of Graded Exercise Therapy (GET) and Cognitive Behavioral Therapy (CBT) were helpful treatments for ME/CFS when compared with Adaptive Pacing Therapy (APT) alone.[24] APT- is effectively Pacing and the Energy Envelope Theory – see *A Path Back to Life* - Chapter 10.

After randomly assigning these 641 people to one of either of these three groups i.e. GET, CBT or APT with outcome assessments taken at 12, 24 and 52 weeks. After analysing the results the PACE researchers concluded GET and CBT were more helpful than APT alone, effectively justifying the then current regimes of GET and CBT.[25]

Specifically, PACE trial researchers reported that these therapies were safe and resulted in recovery for 22% of participants and improvement for 60% to 61%.[26] However, on closer scrutiny the agreed upon definition of improvement had been modified after the results were collated without a clear rationale.[27] These results were therefore rightly questioned by ME/CFS advocate groups and other researchers who asked to see the raw data. The original researchers refused to hand the data over until they were compelled to do so in 2016 after a five-year Freedom of Information campaign!

The patient advocates who obtained the data gave it to another group of researchers to reanalyse. Lo and behold this new analysis revealed some disturbing irregularities. They suggested there were far less benefits, if at all, than originally reported. In particular, they noted that the '**goal posts**,' originally set to define success, were widened significantly **after** the results were obtained (?to give a rosier overall picture?).[28] This is a 'no, no' in any research.

When the data were reanalyzed with the original protocol definition of success goal posts back in place, improvement **decreased by a factor of 3** and recovery rates decreased to 7% for CBT and 4% for GET, not significantly different from controls.[29] Whilst there has not been an official retraction of the original conclusion, the PACE study as it stands is no longer considered reliable.

George Monbiot writing for the Guardian revisited this story and reflected upon its potential relevance to Long COVID. See: https://www.theguardian.com/commentisfree/2021/apr/14/super-spreading-Long COVID-professor-press-coverage

PACE – Doomed before it began?

In order to explore why this study went so wrong, I looked at a PDF of the training manual used to teach the therapists involved in the PACE trial.[30] The first thing that struck me was the impressive effort that had gone into its production. The second was how fatally flawed its education was.[31]

When I looked deeper into its content, it was obvious it lacked the critical understanding we have today, a decade later. Three fundamental things they got wrong were:

1. Therapists were taught the causation of the illness was due to a problem effectively 'all in a person's head' and ongoing symptoms were largely due to deconditioning. (See Chapter 2 - subtitle The Hysteria Myth). Hence, rather than acknowledging an ongoing neurological disease as the WHO had defined this disease to be since the late 1960's, therapists were encouraged to see and therefore to help ME/CFS participants to see, that their symptoms were actually arising from anxiety, intense symptom focusing and/or deconditioning.[32]

2. On the basis of this faulty conclusion regarding the cause of ME/CFS i.e. it's a psychiatric condition, there was no recognition of Chronotropic Intolerance (CI)[33], an autonomic nervous system (ANS) dysfunction that appears to affect at least 9 in 10 people with ME/CFS. This makes heart rate (HR) an unreliable measure of exertion, in my experience for at least the initial three to six months of a rehab program. Due to their belief that ME/CFS was a psychiatric condition, they then incorrectly assumed that rating of perceived exertion (RPE) – See Appendix 3 – utilised effectively by Wallman's study group in WA and my own clinic, was less reliable than heart rate as a monitor.

The PACE researchers therefore did not entertain the possibility that there might be a problem with the autonomic nervous system affecting heart function. At the time of this study a decade ago, this knowledge was only beginning to emerge. Hence, their therapist training manual advised therapists to guide participants more towards heart rate (HR) monitoring than the person's perceived effort (RPE), the opposite that I would now suggest if an autonomic issue was obvious, which it usually is. The patient's perception (RPE) is ultimately the best guide once fear of the process has been dispelled. See *A Path Back to Life* - Chapter 15 Defuse the Loop.

Once a person has reduced their anxiety, the RPE accuracy can then be enhanced, appropriate physical activity individualized and made even safer with heart rate monitoring, which, as I said, in my experience begins to align better with RPE after three to six months of rehab that appears to gently 'kick-start' the autonomic nervous system (ANS) 'engine.'

As I reveal in Chapter 15 in this book, I had CI and if I'd not respected my own perception (RPE) and only taken my heart rate (HR) as a guide, especially in the initial 3 months, I would have crashed within a week. My advice on how to integrate both these measures (RPE and HR) as guides is given in *A Path Back to Life - Chapter 12.*

3. The third troublesome and very practical observation of this practitioner training manual, was the length of the consultations. The initial session was 90-minutes! This was a clear design fault. The first session was meant to serve to explain the rationale behind the program and this was followed by 50-minute weekly sessions! These lengths of time alone would have been very difficult for me and most of the people with ME/CFS that I consulted with to endure, especially when they were at their worst.

Hence, I believe on the grounds of not validating the truth about ME/CFS (i.e. it's a multisystem neurological disease not a psychiatric one), along with the unsuitability for more moderate to severe cases of people with ME/CFS, programs like this have rightly been scrapped and are no longer recommended by NICE or most ME/CFS patient advocate groups around the world.

With the knowledge we have today, however, I believe it would be possible to create an appropriate rehabilitation program like the one I present in the companion book, *A Path Back to Life,* that could be offered and safely researched and refined if necessary. I would expect an individualised rehab program, one whose first principle is that ME/

CFS is a neuro-immune disease, to match the benefits achieved by rehab for other neurological diseases.

Suffice to say, the approach you will be presented with in *A Path Back to Life - The Art of Micro-Rehab*, will be much more like that of the lead US researcher into ME/CFS Dr Nancy Klimas's[34,35] of INIM and Wallman's in Australia, informed by activities that help you unfold your self-awareness, understand and regain trust in your own perceptions (RPE scale) along with the assistance of a heart rate monitor. I believe with our knowledge now of mitochondrial and ANS dysfunction requiring Micro-Rehab, ultra-gentle in its build up in the first three to six months, we can do this safely.

Knowledge is Power

As you might have guessed, I'm making a big deal of explaining this because I have a long history relating to this issue and in order for you, my reader, to not be sent off track by well-meaning practitioners or friends not up to date with the latest approach to safely introducing physical activity, let me arm you with a little personal story that helps to reveal what I believe to be the historic origins of this dilemma.

A Rude Awakening

In 2010 I spoke with the then medical advising doctor to the ME/CFS Association in Australia about some success I was having introducing people with ME/CFS to rehab physical exercise combined in a form I call, the rest/activity dance. *(A Path back to Life- Chapter 14 -15).*

She was interested and agreed that while ME/CFS Australia would not endorse GET, she acknowledged that not all approaches to increasing physical activity were the same and the doctor thought the two stories of patients I'd helped would be a useful contribution.

Knowing the hope these stories could bring to thousands, I spent many hours authoring a detailed piece. Suffice to say I was not happy when it was apparently vetoed by the then board, the presumption being, I was later told, that if exercise had helped my patients, they could not have had ME/CFS!

Hmmm…Really??

Fortunately, times have changed but unfortunately to this day not everyone is aware of this. I'll come back to this conundrum in a moment.

Facing the Demon

So why is the word 'exercise' still so loaded amongst official ME/CFS support groups? I believe this is largely because people with ME/CFS, like myself and members of the board, or their loved-ones have experienced post exertional malaise (PEM) after trying to push through fatigue whilst exercising, then crashing for days or weeks or even relapsing for months. Some of my own and my patients' crashes were self-inflicted, and some occurred due to inappropriate advice by well-meaning but ignorant friends, personal trainers, coaches, gyms and/or other health practitioners.

Let's be clear, these crashes could be severely disabling and frighten one from ever attempting exercise again! Yet, let's also be clear that setbacks can be minimized and as your skills of self-awareness improve; listening/reading your body and applying an RPE and getting familiar with using a heart rate monitor etc., avoided completely.

There is also I believe a deeper group trauma issue at play here. When your struggles are minimized and you are constantly told your dreadful condition is 'all in your head' by medical experts who then tell you that Graded Exercise Therapy (GET) and Cognitive Behavioral Therapy (CBT) are all you need, subtext - "you lazy bugger!" - you are going to kick back!

So, **IF** the ME/CFS support groups mention the word, '*exercise*' in anything but a negative light (even if they do not say Graded Exercise Therapy (GET)), although they may not articulate it, they believe that they would be letting the 'team down' and be seen to be endorsing the older hurtful, incorrect belief as to the cause of this neurological condition, i.e., 'it's just in your head.' Even a sniff of the word 'exercise' is with good reason unacceptable. Right or wrong, this is my understanding of why my article in 2010 demonstrating benefit from appropriate physical activity was rejected.

The Conundrum

This conundrum had bothered me for many years, and it is only now in researching and writing these two books on ME/CFS that I am coming to terms with its understandable origins and am able to articulate a response. Yet, I am also relieved to find others who have realized that dismissing all exercise out of hand, without recognizing its critical role in rehabilitation, is foolish, harmful and potentially dangerous.

For a start, while deconditioning is not the causative factor in ME/CFS it is often the result of it and can be debilitating and ultimately fatal if not treated appropriately. In other words, the illness itself, like other neurological conditions e.g. MS, Parkinson's etc., creates the conditions for deconditioning to occur, unless it is addressed with appropriate physical activity.

The end result of NOT addressing deconditioning can be chronic pain, bone fractures, vertebral disc prolapses, increased risk of falls, gut and heart problems etc. I personally have experienced **all** of these painful complications until I embraced an appropriate ultra-gentle paced rehab exercise regimen that helped pull me out of the ME/CFS quicksand. This will be presented in Chapter 15 and how to implement this in some detail in *A Path Back to Life – The Art of Micro-Rehab*.

In simple terms, as an ex-competitive ping pong player, it helps me to think of this unfolding historical drama like an epic Olympic table-tennis match. On one side of the table we've had the ME/CFS support groups/societies up to date clinicians and biomedical researchers - on the other side of the table we have the Old-Style physicians/psychiatrists (OSPs) stuck on the hysteria hypothesis; both sides digging in. The belief systems being played out are as follows:

Belief Systems OSPs-: Old understanding of cause is that ME/CFS involves primarily severe physical deconditioning following some weird prolonged lazy malingering exercise avoiding personality, which through inactivity creates its own spiral of deconditioning thus perpetuating the condition. In other words, "it's all in your head you lazy bugger!"

*Management – Graded Exercise Therapy (GET) "GET off your bum!" and/or Cognitive Behavioural Therapy (CBT) "Correct Bludging Thoughts!"

Vs

Belief Systems ME/CFS Societies/Biomedical researchers and up to date clinicians -: New understanding of Cause – Neuro-immune condition, with brainstem inflammation, aerobic, autonomic nervous system and immune system dysfunction. The onset most commonly follows a viral infection and can lead to severe debility which in turn leads to secondary problems, including deconditioning. Much like the waxing and waning symptoms of MS, which 60 years ago had also been thought to be 'all in the patient's head,' ME/CFS is also a biomedical neuro-immune disease, NOT a psychiatric problem!

*Management – nobody knows yet i.e., no specific medical treatments, drugs or surgery but definitely ***not*** GET or CBT as this

could be harmful as well as reinforce old, false stereotypes. General measures are recommended, such as pacing and other self-care lifestyle measures and these can make a big difference, where I differ is with the incorporation of 'exercise,' in inverted commas, within a micro-Rehab approach that includes specific mind-body techniques and a method for individualising this approach to ensure safety. See my next book *A Path Back to Life*.

Tragically, in this battle for legitimacy GET and 'any exercise' melded into one and many people with ME/CFS have become too afraid to exert themselves at all. It is sad and ironical that after decades of battling to be recognized as a neurological/biomedical disease not a psychiatric one, when the recognition finally came in 2015, the combatants did not know how to reorient their thinking. Thus, tens-of-thousands of people with ME/CFS continue to have their fears of exercise amplified and consequently suffer due to a **lack of physical activity**.

The fact is **every neurological disorder** known can benefit significantly from a **suitable** level of exercise. Parkinson's disease, Multiple Sclerosis, strokes etc. Exercise has become an invaluable part of their management, being demonstrated to improve function, slow deterioration and even reverse disease. Each condition requires very specific protocols and individualisation to maximise benefit. ME/CFS is no different. It is worth repeating, Dr Klimas's statement addressing people with ME/CFS that headed this chapter:

> *"You must find a way to exercise safely.*
> *If you do not exercise you will get worse."*

How bad can this get? One of my patient's friends who had ME/CFS, Julie, became so exercise averse, bedbound, and deconditioned that one day she got out of bed, stood, and both her legs fractured. This is not a minor issue.

My experience as a patient with ME/CFS and as a treating physician is that if the new understanding of this neuro-immune condition is respected, then carefully introduced rehab that I refer to as Micro-Rehab is invaluable. It is far gentler and more self-directed than any GET trial protocol and can not only reverse deconditioning but positively influence the condition as well.

As Dr Klimas and others have observed, if safely and patiently applied over at least three months, your condition and life will begin to noticeably improve.[36] A three to six-month time frame has been my observation as well.

Given the extensive research confirming we are dealing with a biomedical disorder, perhaps it is time to declare the ping pong match over! There is no longer a need for the OSP's or the ME/CFS groups to be on opposite sides of the table. The condition IS REAL! And yes, just like every other 'Real' neurological disease, appropriately introduced and individualised rehab movement can play an important part in management.

OK I'll say it; "I declare the 'exercise wars' over!"

Chapter 13
Key Points

✓ Graded Exercise Therapy (GET) is no longer recommended by the National Institute for Health and Care Excellence (NICE) as an appropriate therapy for ME/CFS.
✓ There are, however, many other forms and ways of introducing exercise that can be safely undertaken and far from doing harm will help in many ways including

reducing pain, osteoporosis, improving sleep patterns and stamina.

✓ All neurological disorders, including ME/CFS, can receive significant improvement from exercise in the form of paced rehabilitation.

✓ Now that ME/CFS is recognized as a legitimate neurological disease, it's time to declare the exercise wars over and along with all other neurological diseases, get 'rehabing...slowly!'

✓ The companion book, *A Path Back to Life – The Art of Micro-Rehab,* gives detailed suggestions as to how to safely get started.

Chapter 14

EPIGENETIC 'SWITCHES'

"It's not just a matter of playing the genetic cards you're dealt. We have the power to shape our own lives. The reality is a much more optimistic scenario than if it were just a matter of picking the right parents."

JOHN ROWE, PROF OF GERIATRICS AT HARVARD MEDICAL SCHOOL, CHAIRMAN, MACARTHUR FOUNDATION RESEARCH NETWORK ON SUCCESSFUL AGEING.

"Sometimes the greatest scientific breakthroughs happen because someone ignores the prevailing pessimism."

NESSA CAREY, THE EPIGENETICS REVOLUTION: HOW MODERN BIOLOGY IS REWRITING OUR UNDERSTANDING OF GENETICS, DISEASE AND INHERITANCE

How can appropriate lifestyle such as exercise make such a difference to people with a neurological condition like ME/CFS? Epigenetics might give us a clue.

Our Genetic Code

The nature (we were born with) versus nurture (the environment we were raised in) debate about the cause of disease, is undergoing a new revolution. Simply put, until recently many scientists thought the main cause of ill health was written into our DNA code. The code was found to contain a variable sequence of four chemical bases: Adenine, Thymine, Cytosine and Guanine, (abbreviated as A, T, C, G) and was unalterable.

This was the template for the construction of all living things. Two strands of the DNA molecule spiraling together with A lined up across from T, while C formed a complimentary pair with G (see Figure 1).[1]

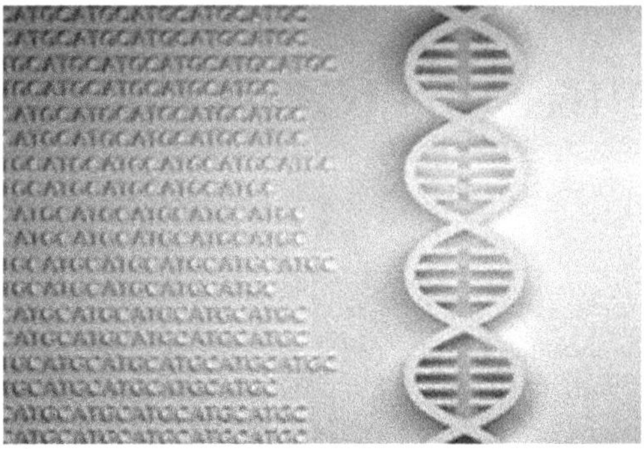

FIG 1 DNA Code

This molecule unzips itself to allow for replication of the DNA or to allow a smaller molecule, messenger ribonucleic acid (mRNA), to read a section of the DNA (i.e. a gene) and translate this into the production of a protein. It then elegantly zips itself up again. So efficient is this molecule that only rarely do errors in replication, known as mutations, occur.[2] In humans, all the information contained within the DNA is compacted into 46 chromosomes (23 pairs) contained within the nucleus of each cell. Half contributed from each of our parents.

It's all in your genes?

The understanding of genes was in its infancy but well underway in Darwin's time at the end of the 19th century. It supported his theory of evolution - random genetic mutations conferring a life-saving advantage or disadvantage to an organism, allowing for the slow process of evolution by natural selection, the so-called 'survival of the fittest.' Yet exactly how genes operated remained a mystery.

When Watson and Crick uncovered the 3D structure of Deoxyribonucleic acid (DNA) and how it functioned over 70 years after Darwin's death, it felt like all had been revealed. It gave a clear mechanism for Darwin's theory. It also came to be associated with the powerful belief that the genetic code you were born with was unchangeable. In other words, your fate was cast in your DNA, a belief so powerful that many of us still hold it, consciously or subconsciously today.

It is important in recovering from ME/CFS to understand that for most illnesses this belief has been debunked, i.e. it is **Not True that our genetic code completely determines our illnesses**. In fact, it only holds true for a few rare diseases (like Thalassemia and Huntington's disease) and it most certainly does not hold true for ME/CFS. Let me explain further.

How our genes CAN change their 'tune'

Genomics, a discipline of genetics, is changing how we view genes. It is involved in sequencing and analyzing the function and structure of genomes, which are the complete set of DNA codes within a single cell of an organism, be they plant, animal or microbe.[3] When the Human Genome Project was completed in the year 2000, it had taken over 10 years to sequence 3 billion genetic chemical base codes at a cost of over 2 billion dollars. (Note: Today, with New Generation Sequencing it takes about a week and now costs closer to $1000 - and falling!).

In the year 2000 the results led to some surprises. Many scientists had predicted the code for producing a human being would contain at least 100,000 genes. In fact, the number was closer to 23,000, a similar number of genes to that found within an earthworm's genome.

Interestingly those 23,000 genes only took up 2% of the DNA found in a human cell. The remaining 98% was labelled 'junk,' in that it was thought to have no function, although it contained startling sequences consistent with our evolutionary past. For example, our most recent evolutionary relatives, the chimpanzee and bonobo monkey, share 99% of the same genetic code as us and believe it or not, a banana shares 60%![4]

What has become increasingly apparent is that which distinguishes us from chimpanzees is not the *number* of genes we have or just the differences in code, but the way in which these genes are being *'played.'* What do I mean?

If we use the analogy of a musical instrument here, let's imagine these 23,000 genes as keys on a very long piano, each key being a **gene**. Most genes in humans contain hundreds or thousands of lined up chemical base codes (A-T; C-G etc. - see Figure 1). This is no ordinary piano, though, some keys would turn out to be tiny (the smallest gene known in humans is 76 bases long and takes less than a second to be read and utilized to make a protein). Others would be huge (the largest known human gene being 2,100,000 bases long and taking 16 hours to be read and utilized to make a muscle protein).

As far as most diseases are concerned, often tens or hundreds of **interacting genes** have been implicated as predisposing us to a singular disease, rather than the idea of one or just a few genes being the cause of each disease, as many thought we would discover.

In addition, it was thought that we were born with a genetic code that couldn't change its tune (i.e. it's expression). Now a branch of genomics, known as the science of epigenetics, (meaning in Greek, 'around the gene') has shown that this is not the case.[5] This is where things become mind-blowing.

Epigenetics

The truth epigenetics has taught us is that our gene's tunes are in constant flux, being influenced by the environment around them. While the template of codes remains the same, they're either being switched off (down-regulated) or switched on (up-regulated). Codes are most commonly downregulated by a biochemical process called methylation that literally covers over parts of the code making that section of our 'musical score' unreadable. Other biochemical processes (e.g. histone modification) switch on or up-regulate certain genes, like those that might cause cancer.

You do not need to fully understand the details, but it turns out this epigenetic flexibility allows individual genes to produce a *variety* of different proteins depending on the environment they find themselves in, healthy or unhealthy.[6,7]

Our understanding grew further with the discovery that the non-coding or 'junk DNA', the non-gene 98%, the rest of the piano and pianist if you like, wasn't junk at all. In fact, it played important structural roles, such as forming the telomere caps to keep our chromosomes (the container for our DNA) from unravelling, as well as a role in 'playing our genes.' Hence, this so-called junk, our deep, past genetic history, was somehow involved in influencing our present and future.

So, *both* the combination of the differences in our genetic code and the complexity of how our 'gene-tunes' (i.e. expression) are played, distinguishes us from the earthworm, chimpanzee and each other. Importantly, **our 'gene-tunes' subtly alter all the time**.

The chemical milieu within each cell is being influenced by the biochemical environment that surrounds it. This in turn is a reflection of what we eat and drink, our social situation, how we feel, think, the air we breathe, the exercise we do or don't do, toxins we might be exposed to, the pills or herbs we swallow, the list goes on. All can affect the biochemical environment and therefore our gene-tunes.

This dynamic interplay between our genes and our world (environment) can make us sick or keep us well. Approximately 90% of our genes are engaged in cooperation with signals from their environment in this way.[8]

Lessons from Twins Confirm Epigenetic Influence

Studying identical (monozygotic) twins, born with a 100% identical genetic code, the closest thing we have to perfect clones, has further illuminated our understanding. Research has been conducted on literally millions of pairs of identical twins and it has been discovered that most diseases and character traits involve nature (our genetic code) and nurture (our environment and choices). As mentioned in Chapter 6 genetic factors do play a role in the development of ME/CFS. This is evidenced by the fact that ME/CFS is significantly more common in identical (55% concordance) than non-identical (19% concordance) twins,.[9-12] But it is not the whole story.

As leading geneticist and twin's researcher, Dr Tim Spector, points out in his very readable book, *Identically Different*, the glaring observation in the identical twin's research is not just the similarities that they possess, but the differences.[13] Pointedly, **more often than not** they *do not* suffer from the same diseases. For instance, if one twin suffers from Rheumatoid Arthritis, a disease with a high level (60-70%) of heritability, in most known populations there's only a 15% chance that the identical twin will also suffer from it.[14]

Taking our understanding of these differences further so that we may learn from them, is a research study that involved 41 identical twin pairs, in which one of the twins developed cancer whilst the other did not.[15] Blood tests looking at DNA methylation sites sought to uncover epigenetic differences between the identical twins. They revealed patterns of difference between the twin who developed cancer and the one who did not. Some of these patterns were present five years prior to the cancer's diagnosis!

This research has helped scientists to hone onto a part of the epigenome relevant to cancer development and could lead to a simple blood screening test for cancer, well before it can be detected by any other means. This could mean earlier treatment with less side effects that may even stop the cancer developing at all.[16] I hope, in time, we will have similar possibilities for ME/CFS and a range of illnesses allowing us to stop them from being triggered in the first place.

Dr Spector concludes: "The most important lesson that we've learned is that you can change your genes, your destiny and that of your children and grandchildren. It really does matter what you do to your body..."[17,18]

While the separation of nature and nurture becomes more blurred, I look forward to future research that uncovers more about the invisible dance between these interplaying factors. While knowing our genetic code (genome) provides us with some useful information about our strengths and weaknesses and some treatments we would be best suited to, knowledge of our epigenome offers huge potential for learning how to 'play' our own code at any given time so that we can be at our healthiest.

Let's be clear, while our personal genome (genetic blueprint), does not change, the way these genes express themselves, our epigenome, can change. This was not known about just 20 years ago. The extent to which this changing of gene expression by our own efforts is possible is beginning to come to light.

For most diseases, including ME/CFS, genes play an important role in predisposing us to them, but often it can be when, where and how we choose to live our lives that will decide whether we will experience illness or not.

How can we influence our gene-tune?

That nurture (diet, love, relationships etc.) can change nature (genetic expression) by influencing it down at its fundamental DNA level is the mind-expanding revelation of epigenetics. Whilst we need to be respectful of the genetic tune we've been dealt, we also need to realize we have a big say in how that tune is played, even when we are already unwell. Let me reiterate, we're not just helpless victims of our genes as so many of us were led to believe.

Scientists and pharmaceutical companies are investigating the possibilities of new medications to alter gene expression. As we understand more about the malfunctioning genes responsible for the problems encountered in ME/CFS, we may discover more effective medical or complementary therapies to treat it.

For now, rather than waiting for these discoveries to happen, there is much we can do for ourselves to rejig the ME/CFS epigenetic pattern to a healthier one. The greatest potential exists in lifestyle changes that might be quite subtle, yet if persisted with, can lift us out of the ME/CFS quicksand as it has done for me and others.

To make the link between our genes and our environment more tangible, let's spend some time looking at some research examples of how lifestyle choices have been shown to affect our epigenetic expression. This will help you to understand how the often seemingly gentle aspects of a holistic lifestyle rehabilitation program can help you in your recovery process from ME/CFS.

Nutrition and our genes (Nutrigenomics)

Here are a few research examples of nutrients that can alter gene expression for the good:[19,20]

Glucosinolates -- found in vegetables such as broccoli, cauliflower and brussel sprouts, activate genes responsible for cleansing the body of toxins.

Lycopene -- found in tomato products, slows down the gene involved in prostate cancer.

Gama-linolenic acid -- found in evening primrose oil, reduces the activity of a gene involved in breast cancer and other malignancies.[21,22]

Focused relaxation and our genes

Tangible beneficial epigenetic effects can occur quite quickly as evidenced by research on the relaxation response (RR). We will look at ways to practice the RR in *A Path Back to Life*. There is much research on the health benefits of regularly practicing focused relaxation or meditation, but for now our interest is in the research of its effects on epigenetics.

In a landmark study published in 2008, 19 healthy long-term RR practitioners were compared with 19 healthy controls who did not practice any form of RR.[23] There were more than 2000 differences in genetic expression found on blood testing between the two groups before the study began. When the 19 controls, who had never practiced RR techniques before, underwent an eight-week relaxation response training course, where they practiced eliciting an RR for 20 minutes each day, their genetic expression profiles changed. Importantly, 433 of the previously differently expressed genes were now shared between the two groups. This study provided the first compelling evidence that the relaxation response elicits specific gene expression changes in just 8-weeks of regular practice.[24]

In a more recent study, blood samples were taken immediately and 15 minutes after an RR session demonstrating epigenetic changes, including reduced inflammation, after just 15 minutes of focused relaxation![25] This confirms that gene expression in at least in certain genes very fluid. In *ME/CFS – A Path Back to Life* I will teach you some of these techniques as part of the rest/activity dance that many people with ME/CFS have found so helpful.

The Power of Lifestyle Change

In terms of the power of healthy lifestyle change to reverse the direction of existing disease via epigenetics, the research of Dr Dean Ornish and colleagues on early prostate cancer has been particularly revealing. Men with early prostate cancer (on watch and wait i.e. not being actively treated yet) who had been randomly assigned to a healthy lifestyle program, not only had a significantly better outcome over five years than those who were not, but showed corresponding significant epigenetic changes.[26,27] Testing of participants revealed that oncogenes, genes that promote cancer, were switched off after just three months on the lifestyle program!

This raises the possibility that cancer, such a feared diagnosis, could be influenced not only by medical therapies, but by the lifestyle choices we make. There are likely to be different lifestyle approaches that are particular for different types of cancer and different individuals. This may well be the beginnings of an explanation as to how so-called spontaneous remissions occur.

In terms of neurological disorders like ME/CFS, there is evidence that people with Multiple Sclerosis (MS) can positively affect the course of their illness by changing their lifestyle.[27-30] In this instance, a five year follow up study found that those people with MS who maintained the prescribed lifestyle changes were actually better on many parameters that had been measured five years earlier.[31] Those who did not maintain the lifestyle changes were worse. As medicos we were taught MS 'naturally' tends to deteriorate year upon year. Perhaps it need not.

While these results are exciting and empowering, as the growing body of research under the banner of Lifestyle Medicine and Mind-body Medicine increases, there is a recognition that one size does not fit all. Different illnesses and individuals within the same illness-grouping may need different individualized lifestyle-treatment plans.[32-36]

Discovering the specific epigenetic triggers, whether they be: a high fever, infection, food, drug, lifestyle, supplement, environmental toxin, etc. that switch on particular diseases, and the food, drug, lifestyle and environmental factors that can switch off these diseases will be the Holy Grail of future research. This will help the doctors of the future to individualize treatment protocols.

Chapter 14
Key Points

✓ The genetic codes we inherited from our parents don't change.

✓ The way our genetic codes express themselves, for better or for worse, can be influenced. This is epigenetics.

✓ Genetic factors do play a role in predisposing us to developing ME/CFS.

✓ The science of Epigenetics suggests it may be possible to recover from ME/CFS by rejigging the way our genetic code expresses itself. At the very least it might provide a mechanism that explains how I and many others with ME/CFS have managed to significantly improve.

Chapter 15

HOPE KNOCKS ON OUR DOOR

"A Journey of 1000 miles begins with a single step."

LAO TZU

The Great Victorian Bike Ride is an annual event in the state of Victoria. In 2004, the hundreds of bike riders enjoying this event passed through Apollo Bay along the Great Ocean Road. Amongst them were Dr Daniel Lewis and his son, Justin. Daniel, a rheumatologist and a friend, had heard I lived in Apollo Bay and phoned to organize a catch up on his way through. During his visit I discovered he had a special interest in rehabilitating people with Fibromyalgia and ME/CFS. It turned out his physiotherapist and yoga teacher off-sider, Laurie Lacey, was soon to holiday in our region and so Daniel organized for him to help me out. Serendipity indeed!

I can still recall Laurie striding up our driveway, his 6ft 8 inches (2 meter) tall frame demonstrating perfect posture. He generously visited daily for a week, walking the 10 km from his campsite to our house to arrive punctually at 10:00 a.m. and guide me through a program. Before we look at this let me paint a brief picture of where I was at back then:

- I barely had the strength to walk down our 10-metre driveway and back.
- I showered second daily because of my lack of energy for it. If I washed my hair, the extra effort involved meant I needed a plastic shower chair to sit on and rest. Then I'd need Tori's help to dry my hair and get dressed before flaking out on the couch for hours recovering.

- Most of my day involved resting on the couch.
- I didn't have the energy to brush my teeth properly so I bought an electric toothbrush.
- To attend any social events, I would rest for days before and then for days after. At the event I would need to sit down frequently and often lie down on a couch or a bed.
- On one occasion Tori dropped me off at the post office and there was an unusually long queue. I was unable to continue standing and embarrassingly had to get someone to get me a chair to sit on, lest I fainted.

ME/CFS in 2004

At this time the Centre for Disease Control in the US believed that ME/CFS was: *'due to such patients harbor mistaken beliefs that they suffer from an actual physical disease. As a result, they remain sedentary out of a misguided fear that activity will make them worse. They then develop severe deconditioning, perpetuating their symptoms.'* [1]

You can see how this would do your head in when you're genuinely ill. I still cringe just reading this, but remember, this was 2004, 11 years before the respected and independent National Academy of Medicine in the US confirmed this to be a 'real' biomedical disease. So much so that they proposed a name change from Chronic Fatigue Syndrome (ME/CFS) to Systemic Exertional Intolerance Disease (SEID) (This name was not adopted as it is, whilst true, too narrow a definition of ME/CFS). [2]

Deconditioning Spiral

In 2004 not even mitochondrial aerobic dysfunction, let alone brainstem inflammation had been confirmed. [3] Like the CDC in the USA, Daniel and Laurie were following the theory that an overanxious stress response and spiraling deconditioning (muscle wasting due to inactivity) was contributing to and/or causing my problems. It made some sense to me too as it was evident in my body. For example, my legs were so thin and weak that I could not stand up from sitting. In order to do so I had to recruit my frail arms to push me up. A recent bone density scan had also shown I had significant osteoporosis.

Apart from restoring muscle and bone condition, Daniel and Laurie also emphasized the need to settle the overactive sympathetic nervous or fight/flight stress system. Laurie's understanding of Yoga was very helpful here.

Yet, while obviously a contributor, I did not believe that the deconditioning theory nor an overactive stress response was the whole answer. It seemed to me to be more of a secondary effect than a primary cause but right then I was desperate, and you don't get a lucky break like this at your door every day! I also respected Daniel and Laurie so that my response to this was essentially, "I don't give a s**t what the theory is, how can I get better?"

Daniel reassured me that while he and Laurie could not be sure of the cause of ME/CFS, they'd had success with their approach, particularly with people with ME/CFS he had admitted to the rehabilitation hospital where they worked in Melbourne. Much as pediatrician, Dr Lionel Lubitz, and his team at the Austin Hospital in Melbourne were having with teenagers with ME/CFS (see Katie's story in *ME/CFS - A Path back to Life*) at that time. However, he was sure with Laurie's assistance and my own and Tori's knowledge and encouragement that I could do this rehab from home. 'But I know how to meditate, and I practiced Yoga and I still got sick!' said a doubting voice in my head.

'Have you got any better ideas?' said another voice inside my head.

It was time to suspend my disbelief and go for it. "Let's do it!" I told Daniel.

If you accept the deconditioning theory and overactive fight/flight stress response to be the complete cause, then the answer to my next question: "How often should I do this program?" would be obvious.

"The more the merrier," would be the answer. We now know that here in lies the saboteur. This is because while people who had severe deconditioning, as I did, due to reasons other than ME/CFS, and are otherwise well, for example, after injuries suffered in a motor vehicle accident, can recover muscle strength and tone within weeks. Exercising daily may be fine for them.

"Daily or as often as feels right to you," answered Daniel, with the wisdom of the day.

Fortunately for me, I intuitively decided to only do the program **every second day and only what I could easily manage**. I told Daniel, "that given I'd had this for 8 years why risk pushing it daily."

The Birth of Micro-Rehab

I now realize this instinct (or was it dumb luck!), was critical to my success. Almost every person with ME/CFS who would consult with me years later told me how exercise had made them worse. They had pushed themselves and tried exercising every day and or too hard, thus incurring the wrath of Post Exertional Malaise (PEM) as a result. The same fate would have awaited me if I'd not reflected upon my previous mistakes, listened in to my instinct and had the confidence to question aspects of the program that had been prescribed for me. So, let's take a closer look at what I actually did as this was the beginnings of what I'd call Micro-Rehab, the focus of my next book: *ME/CFS – A Path Back to Life – The Art of Micro-Rehab*.

Laurie's Program

Laurie introduced me to gentle self-awareness yoga methods, including carefully considered movement and yoga breathing practices (pranayama), something I was familiar with in the past but had let slip. He also introduced me to the Borg rating of perceived effort (RPE) scale with the instruction to **not do any maximal exercise but only submaximal effort of around 6 to 7 out of 10** (See Appendix 3).

Even so, I needed to adjust Laurie's program to begin with to make it much more sensitive to match my situation. I chose to begin at a Borg perceived effort level of 5 and worked my way up slowly from there. **Each person with ME/CFS will be starting from a different point, so do not copy the program outlined below unless supervised to do so** (In *ME/CFS – A Path Back to Life* - I'll give you a safe approach you can try.)

To give you an idea of what this exercise meant for me, I'll describe how I began.

- Yoga breathing exercises (slow belly and alternate nostril breathing for 2 to 5 minutes), gentle stretching once or twice **daily** followed by mindful relaxation twice daily.
- The lightest (yellow) resistance band exercise program **second daily** (never on consecutive days) to increase muscle strength. Laurie suggested starting with 5 reps of the five exercises, I could only manage 2 reps.
- Cycling **(2 or 3 x per week never on consecutive days)** – Using a stationary bike we kept indoors or a foot cycle, I started by slowly rolling my legs on non-resistance band days. The bike was set at its lowest resistance. Laurie had suggested 5 minutes as a starting point. **If I'd done this, I'd have blown the whole program on Day 1!!** Fortunately, I listened to and knew my limitations. This

is crucial to a successful rehabilitation approach to ME/ CFS as we will explore in some detail in the next book. **You must find your own safe starting point and build slowly from there. Mine was just 20 seconds.** My heart rate rose from 40 to 60, by which time I became puffy with a BORG rating of 7 out of ten (see Appendix 3). I then stopped, lay down flat on my back (sometimes with knees bent) with a pillow under my head allowing my breathing to gradually slow and consciously relaxed for 10 minutes using a Yoga Nidra or deep relaxation audio.

- This abnormally slow rise in heart rate with effort, as we looked at in Chapter 11, is known as Chronotropic Intolerance (CI)[4] and is only now being recognized as common in ME/CFS and a reason why one needs to use the RPE scale (1 to 10) and not just a heart rate monitor to judge the aerobic/anaerobic threshold. We'll look at this in detail in *A Path Back to Life – the Art of Micro-Rehab*.

- Initially ALL my rehab activities, be they stretching, strengthening, walking or cycling were guided by the Borg perceived effort scale. This remained the case until the Chronotropic Intolerance eased and my heart rate became congruent with my effort. This took around three months.

I came to call this my **rest/activity dance**, commonly known as pacing but slightly different in its mindful meditative focus and relaxed bodily awareness. Occupational Therapists (OT's) often teach people this concept in effectively managing chronic pain. When I described the approach I had taken to an OT, she called it 'ultra-gentle pacing.' Let me illustrate what I did.

Initially, for each exertion I would rest for at least twice as long or until I felt the exercise was integrated and I was no longer breathless. I overstepped the mark once, early on, before I'd got the hang of not pushing and staying at a sub-maximal level of effort. I was cycling, felt great at the time, so I increased my cycling time by another 30 seconds and cycled faster for this extra time at an 8 out of 10 effort level. I did this after just a week instead of consolidating the previous level for the minimum prescribed time of 2 to 4 weeks before increasing. Post-exertional malaise (PEM) was the result. It freaked me out a bit and knocked my confidence.

As I lay on the coach for most of the day, I reflected upon it and through the pain and brain fog of PEM I eventually forgave myself for my over-enthusiastic transgression. This, along with following Laurie's advice (See Table 1) reduced my recovery time from this PEM episode to three days. Even so, I waited a week, for I can tell you, it took a lot of courage to get back on the bike again, as I feared making the illness worse, as so many people with ME/CFS kept telling me exercise would.

So, the first step was to settle my anxiety. I sat down, took some slow deep belly breaths and did a 5-minute meditation. Then I recalled Laurie's advice and my own techniques for dealing with setbacks (See Table 1):

- I stopped the cycling and resistance band exercises.
- I continued a twice daily yoga breathing, meditation/deep relaxation and gentle stretching regime.
- I recognized some of the Automatic Negative Thoughts (ANT's) that were feeding my fears, like, 'Oh Shit, I've blown it now!' (see Defuse the Loop in *ME/CFS – A Path Back to Life - the Art of Micro-Rehab.*). I also used some of my favorite Positive Emotional Thoughts (PET's) to reassure myself, like, 'I've recovered from setbacks before. Now, at least I know what to do.'
- Importantly, I realized the error I'd made and learnt from it, even though it meant curbing my natural enthusiasm! I needed to work within the faulty aerobic capacity of my mitochondria, even though I didn't know the research at that time. **My thinking was, that like a badly injured muscle, slow careful rehabilitation was the key to rehab my mitochondria**. So, rather than burn all my energy as soon as it rose up, **I saved some in 'the bank.'**
- My incentive was to keep my eyes on a bigger long-term prize, enough energy to sustainably return to life/work again and take the pressure off my loving caring wife. God knows she deserved it. So, whenever the urge to push arose and before each session I'd keep remind myself of what was at stake.

Table 1 Strategies for Facing Setbacks

These strategies combined to help me to defuse my anxiety. So, once I felt ready, I reinstated strength work and cycling at half the level I had reached prior to this setback, for the next week, before gradually increasing again by 15 seconds and staying at this new safe level for the next 2 to 4 weeks, before increasing by another 15 seconds.

If I felt poorly on an exercise day I would either halve the amount just for that session or skip it that day focusing more on just the breathing exercises, gentle stretching, relaxation and meditation. I made sure I did something.

I learnt Laurie was right. To rehabilitate safely through careful self-monitoring, I had to keep my maximum effort level at about 2/3rds (i.e. 6-7/10 on the Borg RPE scale -see Appendix 3). As I progressed, I continued to be attentive to staying in the 6 to 7/10 range, and eventually, as a back-up check, was able to see that this corresponded with keeping my heart rate below 110 to avoid a crash (I wore a heart-rate monitor). As I said, the CI seemed to largely resolve itself after three months of this rehab approach. This suggests that my Autonomic Nervous System was rehabilitating.

I also discovered that if my legs became particularly sore whilst cycling on our stationary bike, I could simply stop, remain seated on the bike, deepen my breathing so as to draw in extra oxygen and wait until the soreness settled, which would usually only take 30 to 60 seconds. I would then *increase* the bike's resistance setting slightly and slowly recommence, repeating this pattern if necessary. This helped to increase my leg strength. If the leg pain did not settle within 60 seconds of resting with slow belly breathing, I would discontinue the cycling session, hydrate and lie down with my feet elevated (a cushion beneath them) and actively relax for 10 minutes with a Yoga Nidra (a deep guided relaxation).

As the weeks went by, I found that I needed less and less rest time to integrate the rehab activity and feel ready to move again. Without over-exerting myself, I was able to consolidate a new level of 3-pronged activity (stretching, resistance bands, stationary cycling) every 2 to 4 weeks and hence increase my program activity level at least once or twice a month.

Some of you might see this as a painstaking approach. In some ways it is, but after I had tried so many things over 8 years, including expensive alternative therapies and was watching Tori buckling under the weight of being my carer without her family's support, I would have tried just about anything to improve our situation. Besides, what did I have to lose, I had lots of time to apply myself and it gave me hope.

I timetabled these sessions as a priority, making sure to minimize or exclude other activities, like washing my hair on aerobic (cycling session) days, and kept a journal of my progress. After about three months on this regime, I felt my energy lift and I was able to achieve so much more each day. I could also now rise from sitting using my thigh muscles alone again. Yay!

I now realize that the regular defusing of my anxiety (the rest part of the rest-activity dance) using deep slow belly breathing, alternate nostril breathing, meditation, Yoga Nidra and replacing ANTs with PETs, was just as important as the 3-pronged activity part of the dance.

Laurie also taught me another yoga breathing technique, 'bellows breathing,' but I found this was too strong for me, causing stomach pain, so I left this out of my regime.

My realization then, as with my earlier decision to do a full program of Rehab every second day not daily, was that while Daniel and Laurie gave me a range of potentially useful tools to assist in my rehabilitation, and I would have loved to have just been told what to do and just have done it, it was up to me to learn to **read** my body's signals and guide myself.

This happened best when I relaxed. Through a clearer less anxious mind and without pushing to meet some timetable, I began to see tiny bits of progress and my confidence grew. Still, this thrill too could have set me back, so with bigger aims to try for I encouraged myself to hold steady and not get over-excited with each small gain. Saving energy in the bank until there was enough there to restore itself, not spending it all at once was difficult but critical to me getting a fuller life back.

At four months I was able to walk outside on the footpath with others. All the while I was able to maintain a non-anxious awareness of whether my body was needing a rest or not. To start with I walked one house length away from our place and back second daily, increasing by one house every two to four weeks. It felt so good to be outside without intense fear. If my body said it was tired, I would thank it for its message and respond to its call by slowing or stopping for a minute or two. I knew where all the low fences or bus stops were where I could sit for a bit if I needed to.

By 10 months I was able to walk the one kilometer into the township, without needing to stop for a rest, sit with a friend for a cuppa in a cafe, then walk home, again, without stopping to rest. I would then lie down for 10 minutes and do a Yoga Nidra (deep muscle relaxation) followed by a 10-minute meditation and I'd feel ready to tackle the rest of the day.

It was like I'd been driving a broken-down manual car that for 8 years that had been inconsistently, and rarely, making it out of neutral or first gear and too often going into reverse with PEM. Kick starting to second gear and comfortably staying there for most of the day was incredible!

Let me clarify, I still had to be careful not to push into third, fourth or fifth gear, that is to say, my energy levels were still well below that of a healthy person, like Tori, but were **100** times higher than they had been prior to commencing the program. I felt like, after eight years, I'd been released from a low-energy prison. It felt amazing! I had a chance to expand my life again and I was so grateful for this.

New Opportunities

After my father, Lee's death, my mother, Rachel, began to see the truth of our struggles and her generosity allowed us to move to the city of Geelong and purchase a house in which we could both live and work. Her support and the serendipitous intervention of Daniel and Laurie helped me regain enough physical and emotional strength to attempt a return to some part-time work for the first time in 11 years.

We had good friends in Geelong, and they put us onto a reliable builder, who refitted our newly acquired house, allowing us to shut off our clinic from our living area. A new coat of paint and brass plaques at the front entrance set the scene for a new beginning.

Tori and I had a room each in which we could work simultaneously, both playing the role of receptionist as needed. Working from home would also allow me to, if necessary, adjust my appointment times and rest in between seeing people. I was nervous and excited about returning to work. Not working, regardless of the reason, had been demoralizing and this was a set up I felt I could handle.

In addition, I was passionate about helping people affected by ME/CFS. The Geelong Division of General Practice (later called Medicare Local) was very supportive and advertised my availability for this role to the other GPs in the region. I also met with the local ME/CFS support group. By March 2007, I was ready to go. It felt like a monumental step and I was so grateful for the opportunity to work once again, especially to be able to help people who had been affected by ME/CFS as I had been.

My return to work took other forms as well. Between 2007 and 2012, in addition to my clinical work I produced a stress management CD, teaching meditation and relaxation skills (see www.drstevensommer. com), and was given the opportunity to return to medical teaching. This took the form of a lecture and tutorial series for first year medical students on self-care and stress management at Deakin University Medical School. AstraZeneca, a pharmaceutical company, also employed me to present sessions on self-care for general practitioners. Life was looking up again.

Chapter 15
Key Points

✓ ME/CFS can strike slowly or suddenly. It can affect people across all socio-economic groups and cultures.

✓ I discovered that when you can no longer trust your body to cope with situations you previously found easy to deal with, everyday life becomes a challenge. For me and so many others battling this debilitating illness, post-exertional malaise (PEM), a cardinal feature of the condition, meant crashes into flu-like fatigue for days after minimal overexertion. This made active participation, both social and in a work role nigh on impossible.

✓ In 2004 the theory as to the presumed cause and treatment of ME/CFS blurred together and were thought to be related to spiraling deconditioning and an over-sensitive anxious response.

✓ More recent research recognizes ME/CFS as a biomedical disorder with dysfunctional aerobic metabolism within mitochondria (the energy batteries of our cells), multiple dysfunctional immune system parameters, autonomic nervous system (ANS) dystonia and a range of other problems, including inflammation in the brainstem. See Chapter 12 Summary Table.

✓ How did I recover enough to be able to return to work? Improved social and financial support from my family and the serendipitous knock on our door of Dr Daniel Lewis and Laurie Lacey. Apart from my determination to have a go, their contact and assistance would be the key beginnings of what became my understanding of the holistic and Micro-Rehab approach that over a five-year period, I shared with people with ME/CFS who sought my help in our clinic. I present this in detail, including stories from our patients, in *A Path Back to Life- the Art of Micro-Rehab*.

✓ In Table 1 I share the strategies I used to deal with any setbacks.

EPILOGUE

I managed to track down Chris (see Chapter 1), thirty years on from our first meeting. His wife, Louisa, continues to teach, Charlotte is married and working as a nurse and Mark is a manager at a local fast-food chain. It took Chris till 2002 (13 years), but he managed to return to part-time work. He still has to be careful though; he aims to get to bed before 10.00pm every night and paces things carefully.

When I inquired as to what he'd found most helpful for improving his experience of ME/CFS, apart from the passing of time, there were three standouts. When his wife Louisa's mother died in the year 2000, they received an inheritance and paid off their mortgage, which relieved the family's financial burdens. Financial pressures had weighed heavily on Chris's mental health as Louisa had carried the full responsibility for the family's finances for years. Without this pressure he'd been able to focus in more on his own needs. He joined a hospital outpatient rehab program for ME/CFS and two years later felt able to apply for and handle part-time security work again.

Second was applying pacing principles that he'd learnt from an online course. Third was getting off refined sugar and sticking to an 'avoid-white's' diet that a naturopath had placed him on. He really notices after an initial boost his energy drops if he eats/drinks (high GI) sweet things and so avoids these.

❦

A Twist in the Tale

I may not have had answers for Chris in 1989, but when I did, running an ME/CFS clinic was both challenging and rewarding. Hearing the difficulties my patients were facing was at times heartbreaking, whilst on the other hand, seeing them benefit from the strategies I was teaching was gratifying. While the vast majority were on a journey of life-restoration my own journey was becoming a lot more complicated. You see, while my patients' improvements were growing, I was developing new persistent symptoms. The development of another illness needed to be considered.

New Challenges

In 2009 I was diagnosed with Parkinson's Disease (PD), another neurological illness, one my father and his sister (my aunt) had had. When Crohn's disease and Grave's disease followed in quick succession, I was hospitalized on four separate occasions, lost near to 20kg in weight, and experienced life-threatening situations. I also had severe multiple drug intolerances just as I'd had with ME/CFS. I had to accept, once again, I was too unwell to continue working. In October 2011, after 5 years, Tori and my clinic for people diagnosed with ME/CFS closed its doors.

Another eight-year battle followed. This battle was won thanks to: radiation treatment to ablate the thyroid gland and thus abate Grave's disease, an intravenous biologic medication (Infliximab) for Crohn's disease, successful Deep Brain Stimulation (DBS) brain surgery for Parkinson's along with a heart pacemaker. I'd had six mini-strokes, Transient Ischemic Attacks (TIA's), from low blood pressure where I'd lost the ability to speak intelligibly for around five minutes at a time. My legs were also swelling due to cardiac failure; fortunately this all resolved with the heart pacemaker.

Without Tori by my side the whole way I would not have survived to tell this tale.

I now have a new lease on life that Tori and I are enjoying. So much so that in 2022 I plan a return to public speaking and lecturing, something

I enjoy. Researching and writing this book has been a purposeful part of this renaissance in my health. In 2019 I was invited to become a member of the Medical Advisory Committee of Emerge Australia, the main ME/CFS Society in Australia.

Let me finish by reiterating that the majority of people with ME/CFS will **not** develop Grave's, Parkinson's or Crohn's disease as I did. However, it has been reported in a study involving 960 people with ME/CFS attending four clinics specializing in treating this disease that 84% had co-morbidities,[1] so it's important to be aware that ME/CFS can coexist with other illnesses or can be the herald of another illness, sometimes years in advance (See Appendix 4). For example, one of the people I consulted with who'd been diagnosed with ME/CFS ended up developing Multiple Sclerosis a year later. The take home message? If new and/or persistent symptoms develop, make sure you check them out with your doctor.

❦

For those interested in learning more about my biography, see my book, *Finding Hope,* and my relaxation/meditation audio, *Restoring Balance* at www.drstevensommer.com.

APPENDIX 1

ME/CFS CANADIAN CLINICAL DIAGNOSTIC CRITERIA SUMMARY

To diagnose ME/CFS the patient must have the following:

- Pathological fatigue, post-exertional malaise, sleep problems, pain, two neurocognitive symptoms, and at least one symptom from two of the following categories: autonomic, neuroendocrine, immune.
- The fatigue and the other symptoms must persist, or be relapsing for at least six months in adults, or three months in children. A provisional diagnosis may be possible earlier.
- The symptoms cannot be explained by another illness.

Improved diagnostic accuracy can be obtained by measuring the severity and frequency of the listed symptoms**

Symptoms	Description of Symptoms
1 (a) **Pathological fatigue**	A significant degree of new onset, unexplained, persistent or recurrent physical and/or mental fatigue that substantially reduces activity levels and which is not the result of ongoing exertion and not relieved by rest.
(b) **Post-exertional malaise**	Mild exertion or even normal activities followed by malaise: the loss of physical and mental stamina and/or worsening of other symptoms. Recovery is delayed, taking more than 24 hours.

(c) **Stress** of any kind can aggravate symptoms.

2. **Sleep problems**	Sleep is un-refreshing: disturbed quantity - daytime hypersomnia or night-time insomnia and/or disturbed rhythm – day/night reversal. Rarely is there no sleep problem.
3. **Pain**	Pain is widespread, migratory or localized: Myalgia; arthralgia (without signs of inflammation); and/or headache - a new type, pattern or severity. Rarely is there no pain.
4. **Neurological/ Cognitive Manifestations**	(Two Neurocognitive symptoms) impaired concentration, short term memory or word retrieval; hypersensitivity to light, noise or emotional overload; confusion; disorientation; slowness of thought; muscle weakness; ataxia.

At least one symptom from two of these categories:

5. (a) **Autonomic**	Orthostatic intolerance: neurally mediated hypotension (NMH); postural orthostatic tachycardia (POTS); light headedness; extreme pallor; palpitations; exertional shortness of breath; urinary frequency; irritable bowel syndrome (lBS); nausea.
(b) **Neuroendocrine**	low body temperature; cold extremities; sweating; intolerance to heat or cold; reduced tolerance for stress; other symptoms worsen with stress; weight change; abnormal appetite.
(c) **Immune**	recurrent flu-like symptoms; sore throats; tender lymph nodes; fevers; new sensitivities to food, medicines, odors or chemicals.

6. The illness **persists** for at least 6 months in adults or 3 months in children.

For doctors - Canadian Clinical Criteria Summary - http://saME/CFS. asn.au/download/consensus_overview_me_ME/CFS.pdf   (accessed March 2019)

http://www.me-de-patienten.nl/CCC   Checklist.pdf   (accessed March 2019)

APPENDIX 2

OTHER POTENTIAL DIAGNOSES (DIFFERENTIAL DX)

Conditions that may mimic or can coexist with ME/CFS (alphabetically listed):

- Adrenal Insufficiency
- Anemia
- Cancer
- Celiac
- Chronic Viral infections e.g. EBV, CMV, hepatitis, HIV/AIDS
- Cranio-cervical Instability/Atlantoaxial instability (More common in Ehler's Danlos Syndrome & Downs Syndrome).
- Diabetes Mellitus
- Fibromyalgia
- Hypothyroidism
- Heavy metal toxicity (proven by urine or hair analysis)
- Lyme Disease and other Rickettsial infections
- Multiple Sclerosis
- Orthostatic Hypotension
- Parkinson's disease (early)
- Polymyalgia Rheumatica
- Postural Orthostatic Tachycardia syndrome (POTS)
- Psychiatric disorders – anxiety depression, eating disorders (anorexia nervosa, bulemia)
- Rheumatological diseases eg. Rheumatoid Arthritis, Lupus, Polymyalgia Rheumatica, Sjogren's Syndrome, Marfans Syndrome, Ehlers Danlos Syndrome
- Sinoatrial node dysfunction leading to bradycardia (slow

heart rate)
- Sleep Disorders – Sleep Apnea, Restless Legs Syndrome
- Supplementation or medication side effect or interaction

These conditions may give you symptoms with similarities to ME/CFS, including severe fatigue, and may need to be excluded (see link below) by a thorough medical history, examination and medical testing.

https://emedicine.medscape.com/article/235980-differential

APPENDIX 3

RATING OF PERCEIVED EXERTION (RPE) SCALE

Modified Borg Rating of Perceived Exertion (Borg RPE) scale[1]

1-2   No effort at all

2-3   Minimal effort

3-4   Extremely light effort

4-5   Very Light (e.g. walking slowly at your own pace)

5-6   Light

6-7   Somewhat hard. You start to huff & puff but can still conduct a conversation if needs be. (You feel OK to continue, YET – this is where I suggest you stop initially (i.e. the first 3 months) and mindfully rest, so you can bank the benefit and build resilience.)

7-8   Hard

8-9   Very Hard

10   Maximal exertion

Note: The original Borg Scale was 6 to 20.

---

1   http://www.cdc.gov/physicalactivity/basics/measuring/exertion.htm (accessed June 2020)

APPENDIX 4

CONDITIONS THAT COMMONLY CO-EXIST WITH ME/CFS

(Co-morbitities) Modified from Bateman et al[1]

Autonomic Nervous System
Orthostatic Hypotension, POTS, NMH

Rheumatological
Fibromyalgia, Ehlers Danlos Syndrome, Temperomandibular (Jaw) Joint (TMJ) Dysfunction, Sicca Syndrome (dry mucous membranes)

Gastrointestinal
Food allergies and intolerances, Irritable Bowel Syndrome (IBS), Coeliac disease, gut motility problems e.g with the migratory motor complex, Small Intestinal Bowel Overgrowth (SIBO)

Neurological
Sensory hypersensitivities (e.g. to noise, bright lights), poor balance, migraines, peripheral neuropathy.

Endocrine /Metabolic
Hypothyroidism, HPA axis dysfunction, Metabolic Syndrome

Immunological Disorders
Worsened Allergies, Mast Cell Activation Syndrome, Multiple Chemical Sensitivities Chronic infections, Immunodeficiencies

---

1   Bateman L, Bested A C, Bonilla H F, et al. Myalgic Encephalomyelitis/Chronic Fatigue Syndrome: Essentials of Diagnosis and Management. Mayo Clinic Proceedings Consensus Recommendations. Open Access August 25, 2021; TABLE 3. DOI:https//doi.org/10.1016/j.mayocp.2021.07.004 full text link: Read it here

Sleep Disorders
Sleep apnoea, restless leg syndrome, periodic limb movement disorder

Psychiatric Disorders
Secondary anxiety, secondary depression

Gynaecological Disorders
Endometriosis, premenstrual syndrome, vulvodynia

Miscellaneous
Interstitial cystitis, overactive bladder, nutritional deficiencies (e.g. vitamin B12, D), obesity, underweight.

ABOUT THE AUTHORS

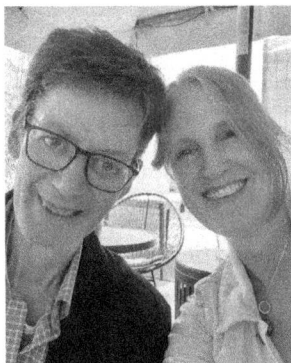

Steven Sommer M.B.,B.S FRACGP

Steven graduated from Monash University Medical School in 1984. He then worked in hospital settings over 4 years, before successfully completing his general practice training to become a Fellow of the Royal Australian College of General Practitioners in 1991.

He developed a special interest in mindfulness-based stress management in the early 90's whilst working as a GP and senior lecturer at Monash University's Department of General Practice and he was an invited Grand Round presenter on this topic at several major teaching hospitals.

In 1993 he took on the role of president of the Whole Health Institute of Australasia (WHI); a non-profit educational organization. In 1996 his health collapsed; he was eventually diagnosed with ME/CFS and too unwell to continue, he had to relinquish all his previous roles.

It took 11 years, but by 2007 he'd found a way to recover enough from ME/CFS to return to general practice and teaching at Deakin University Medical School. However, further health crises in 2011, unrelated to ME/CFS (Parkinson's, Graves and Crohn's disease) left him unable to continue as a practitioner. This has opened a space for him to research and share his ideas and insights through his writing. This is the first of two books he's authored on ME/CFS, *A Path Back to Life* being the second.

His first book, Finding Hope (2017), was well-received. (see wwwdrstevensommer.com).

In 2019 Steven was invited and joined the inaugural Medical Advisory Committee for Emerge (ME/CFS) Australia.

Tori Sommer B.App.Sc.(Chiro), BA(psych).

After completing her BA(psych) at Melbourne University, Tori worked and travelled through Europe for 2 years before returning to five more years of study at the Royal Melbourne Institute of technology (RMIT) to become a chiropractor. During her chiropractic studies she joined the Whole Health Institute (WHI) and headed up the student committee. Her interest in performing and singing led her to meeting Steven. They met on stage as part of the WHI comedy troupe performing at a student healthcare conference in 1991.

Tori worked and ran her own clinic as a chiropractor until 2011 when her energies were needed to care full time for Steven. Over these difficult years she has found solace in exploring her interests and developing her skills in the Arts, including children's book illustration. She has been accepted to complete an honors degree in Visual Arts at Deakin University in Geelong.

Steven and Tori recently celebrated 27 years of marriage. They live in Geelong together with their three cats, Princess Pippy (Pip), and Tooley Scrumptious (Scrumps) and Mr. Pye Pye.

REFERENCES

Introduction

1. Sommer SJ. Finding Hope - when facing serious disease. Inspiring Stories, Healing Insights and Health Research. Amazon.com 2017.
2. Ibid p 237

Chapter 1 ME/CFS 1989 Chris's Story

Chapter 2 A Brief History of ME/CFS

1. https://www.a4medicine.co.uk/chronic-fatigue-syndrome-ME/CFS/
2. Darwin's Illness Revisited. BMJ 2009; 339 doi: https://doi.org/10.1136/bmj.b4968 (Published 14 December 2009) Cite this as: BMJ 2009;339:b4968
3. https://en.wikipedia.org/wiki/Florence_Nightingale
4. McIntyre, A, M.E.- Chronic Fatigue Syndrome: a practical guide. Thorsons, London 1998:1-33.
5. Ibid
6. Ibid
7. https://www.mayoclinic.org/diseases-conditions/polio/symptoms-causes/syc-20376512
8. https://www1.racgp.org.au/newsgp/clinical/what-are-the-long-term-health-risks-post-covid-19
9. Ramsay AM, Post Viral Fatigue Syndrome: The Saga of Royal Free Disease. Gower Medical Publishing 1988:12.
10. McEvedy CP, Beard AW, Concept of benign myalgic encephalömyelitis. Br Med J; 1 1967:11-15.
11. http:/www.independent.co.uk/news/orbituaries-colin-mcevedy-8715136.html

Chapter 3 Diagnosis, Prevalence and Prognosis

1. https://www.who.int/classifications/icd/en/
2. Twisk FNM. Myalgic Encephalomyelitis, Chronic Fatigue Syndrome, and Chronic Fatigue: Three Distinct Entities Requiring Complete Different Approaches. Curr Rheumatol Rep. 2019 May 9;21(6):27. doi: 10.1007/s11926-019-0823-z. Review.
3. Bateman L, Bested A C, Bonilla HF, et al. Myalgic Encephalomyelitis/Chronic Fatigue Syndrome: Essentials of Diagnosis and Management. Mayo Clinic Proceedings Consensus Recommendations. Open Access August 25, 2021.
4. DOI:https//doi.org/10.1016/j.mayocp.2021.07.004 see link: Read it here
5. US Institute of Medicine. Beyond Myalgic Encephalomyelitis/Chronic Fatigue Syndrome: Redefining an Illness. Washington, DC: The National Academies Press; 2015.https://doi.org/10.17226/19012
6. Darbishire L, Risdale L, Seed P T. Distinguishing patients with chronic fatigue with those with Chronic Fatigue Syndrome: a diagnostic study in UK primary care. Br J Gen Pract 2003;53(491):441-445.
7. Clauw DJ. Perspectives on fatigue from the study of chronic fatigue syndrome and related conditions. PM&R 2010; 2 (5): 414-430.

8. Walitt B, Ceko M, Gracely JL, Gracely RH. Neuroimaging of Central Sensitivity Syndromes: Key Insights from the Scientific Literature. Curr Rheumatol Rev. 2016;12(1):55-87.
9. Ibid 3
10. Bateman L, Darakjy S, Klimas N,et al.Chronic fatigue syndrome and co-morbid and consequent conditions: evidence from a multi-site clinical epidemiology study. Fatigue. 2015; 3:1-15.
11. Caruthers BA, van de Sande MI. Myalgic Encephalomyelitis: A Clinical Case definition ad Guidelines for Medical Practitioners. An Overview of the Canadian Consensus Document.
12. Darbishire L, Ridsdale L, Seed PT. Distinguishing patients with chronic fatigue from those with chronic fatigue syndrome: a diagnostic study in UK primary care. Br J Gen Pract. 2003;53(491):441-445.
13. Dolezal B A, Neufeld EV, Boland D M, et al. Interrelationship between sleep and exercise: a systematic review [erratum appears in Adv Prev Med. 2017;2017:5979510]. Adv Prev Med. 2017; 2017: 1364387
14. Hearing C M, Chang W C, Szuhany K L , et al. Physical exercise for treatment of mood disorders: a critical review. Curr Behav Neurosci Rep. 2016; 3: 350-359
15. Geneen L J, Moore R A, Clarke C, et al. Physical activity and exercise for chronic pain in adults: an overview of Cochrane Reviews. Cochrane Database Syst Rev. 2017; 2017: CD011279
16. Godman H. Regular exercise changes the brain to improve memory, thinking skills. Harvard Health Blog. April 2014 https://www.health.harvard.edu/blog/regular-exercise-changes-brain-improve-memory-thinking-skills-201404097110
17. Van Oosterwijck J. Nijs J. Meeus M, et al. Pain inhibition and postexertional malaise in myalgic encephalomyelitis/chronic fatigue syndrome: an experimental study. J Intern ed. 2010; 268: 265-278 View in Article
18. Cook D B, Light A R, Light K C, et al. Neural consequences of post-exertion malaise in myalgic encephalomyelitis/chronic fatigue syndrome. Brain Behav Immun. 2017; 62: 87-99 View in Article
19. Nijs J., Van Oosterwijck J., Meeus M., Lambrecht L., Metzger K., Frémont M., Paul L. Unravelling the nature of postexertional malaise in myalgic encephalomyelitis/chronic fatigue syndrome: the role of elastase, complement C4a and interleukin-1beta. J. Intern. Med. 2010;267(4):418–435. doi: 10.1111/j.1365-2796.2009.02178.x.
20. VanNess J.M., Stevens S.R., Bateman L., Stiles T.L., Snell C.R. Postexertional malaise in women with chronic fatigue syndrome. J. Womens Health (Larchmt) 2010;19(2):239–244.
21. Jasona LA, Zinn ML, Zinn MA. Myalgic Encephalomyelitis: Symptoms and Biomarkers Curr Neuropharmacol. 2015 Sep; 13(5): 701–734.
22. Ibid
23. Rowe P. General information brochure on orthostatic intolerance and its treatment. March 2014. See: https://www.dysautonomiainternational.org/pdf/RoweOIsummary.pdf
24. Ocon A J, Messer Z R, Medow M S, et al. Increasing orthostatic stress impairs neurocognitive functioning in chronic fatigue syndrome with postural tachycardia syndrome. Clin Sci (Lond). 2012; 122: 227-238.
25. Dani M, Dirksken A, Taraborrelli P, et al. Autonomic dysfunction in 'long COVID': rationale, physiology and management strategies. Clin Med (Lond). 2021 Jan; 21(1): e63–e67.
26. Ibid

27.   Potential Melastatin 3 Ion Channel Activity in Natural Killer Cells From Chronic Fatigue Syndrome/ Myalgic Encephalomyelitis Patients. Mol Med. 2019 Apr 23;25(1):14.

28.   Hornig M, MOntoya JG, Klimas NG, Levine S, Felsenstein D, et al. Distinct plasma immune signatures in ME/CFS are present early in the course of illness. Sci Adv 2015;1:e1400121.

29.   Bakken I, Tveito K, et al. Two age peaks in the incidence of chronic fatigue syndrome/ myalgic encephalomyelitis: a population-based registry from Norway 2008-2012. BMC Medicine 2014 Oct:12;167.

30.   US Institute of Medicine Beyond Myalgic Encephalomyelitis/Chronic Fatigue Syndrome: Redefining an Illness. Washington, DC: The National Academies Press; 2015.https://doi.org/10.17226/19012

31.   Johnston SC, Staines DR, Marshall-Gradisnik SM. Epidemiological characteristics of chronic fatigue syndrome/myalgic encephalomyelitis in Australian Patients. Clinical Epidemiology; 2016 May;8:97-107.

32.   Jason L.A., Porter N., Brown M. ME/CFS: a review of epidemiology and natural history studies. Bull IAME/CFS ME. 2009;17(3):88–106.

33.   Hamaguchi M., Kawahito Y., Takeda N., Kato T., Kojima T. Characteristics of chronic fatigue syndrome in a Japanese community population: chronic fatigue syndrome in Japan. Clin Rheumatol. 2011;30(7):895–906.

34.   Kim C.H., Shin H.C., Won C.W. Prevalence of chronic fatigue and chronic fatigue syndrome in Korea: community-based primary care study. J Korean Med Sci. 2005;20(4):529–534.

35.   Lindal E., Stefánsson J.G., Bergmann S. The prevalence of chronic fatigue syndrome in Iceland—a national comparison by gender drawing on four different criteria. Nord J Psychiatry. 2002;56(4):273–277. [published correction appears in Nord J Psychiatry. 2006;60(?):183]

36.   Njoku M.G., Jason L.A., Torres-Harding S.R. The prevalence of chronic fatigue syndrome in Nigeria. J Health Psychol. 2007;12(3):461–474.

37.   Reyes M., Nisenbaum R., Hoaglin D.C. Prevalence and incidence of chronic fatigue syndrome in Wichita, Kansas. Arch Intern Med. 2003;163(13):1530–1536.

38.   Reynolds KJ, Vernon SD, Bouchery E, Reeves WC. The economic impact of chronic fatigue syndrome. Cost Effect Res Alloc 2004;2:4.

39.   Cairns RH. Systematic review describing the prognosis of chronic fatigue syndrome. Occup Med (Oxford, England) 2005;55(1):20–31.

40.   March D. The Natural Course of Chronic Fatigue Syndrome: Evidence from a Multi-Site Clinical Epidemiology Study. Presentation IAME/CFS San Francisco Conference 2014.

41.   https://www.betterhealth.vic.gov.au/health/conditionsandtreatments/chronic-fatigue-syndrome-ME/CFS [accessed March 2020]

42.   Brown MM, Bell DS, Jason LA, Christos C, Bell DE. Understanding long-term outcomes of chronic fatigue syndrome. J Clin Psychol 2012;68(9):1028–35.

43.   Joyce J, Hotopf M, Wessely S. The prognosis of chronic fatigue and chronic fatigue syndrome: a systematic review. Q J Med 1997;90(3):223–33.

44.   Ibid

45.   Nisenbaum R, Jones A, Jones J, Reeves W. Longitudinal analysis of symptoms reported by patients with chronic fatigue syndrome. Ann Epi 2000;10(7):458.

46.   Ciccone DS, Chandler HK, Natelson BH. Illness trajectories in the chronic fatigue syndrome: a longitudinal study of improvers versus non-improvers. J Nerv Ment Dis

2010;198(7):486–93.

47. Ibid 3

48. Pheby D, Saffron L. Risk factors for severe ME/CFS. Biol Med 2009;1(4):50–74.

49. Bell DS. Twenty-five year follow-up in chronic fatigue syndrome: Rising Incapacity. Mass CFIDS Assoc. Continuing Education Lecture April 16, 2011.

50. Collin Sm, Crawley E. Specialist treatment for chronic fatigue syndrome/ME: a cohort study amongst adult patients in the UK. BMC Health Services Research.2017 July;17(1):488.

51. Cox D L, Findley L J. The management of chronic fatigue syndrome in an inpatient setting: presentation of an approach and perceived outcome. Br J Occup Ther. 1998; 61: 405-409.

52. Unger E.R. Lin J.-M.S.Tian H.et al.Multi-site clinical assessment of myalgic encephalomyelitis/chronic fatigue syndrome (MCAM): design and implementation of a prospective/retrospective rolling cohort study Am J Epidemiol. 2017; 185: 617-626

53. [erratum appears in Am J Epidemiol. 2017;186(1):129].

54. Pendergrast T, Brown A, Sunnquist M, et al. Housebound versus non-housebound patients with myalgic encephalomyelitis and chronic fatigue syndrome. Chronic Illn. 2016; 12: 292-307.

55. The voice of the patient. A series of reports from the U.S. Food and Drug Administration's (FDA's) patient-focused drug development initiative. September 2013.https://www.fda.gov/downloads/forindustry/userfees/prescriptiondruguserfee/ucm368806.pdf [Accessed: December 2020]

56. Rusu C, Gee ME, Lagacé C, Parlor M. Chronic fatigue syndrome and fibromyalgia in Canada: prevalence and associations with six health status indicators. Health Prom Chron Dis Prev Can 2015;35(1):3–11.

57. Taylor RR, Kielhofner GW. Work-related impairment and employment-focused rehabilitation options for individuals with chronic fatigue syndrome: A review. J Mental Health 2005;14(3):253–267.

58. Crawley EM, Emond AM, Sterne JAC. Unidentified chronic fatigue syndrome/ myalgic encephalomyelitis (ME/CFS/ME) is a major cause of school absence: surveillance outcomes from school-based clinics. BMJ Open 2011;1(2):e000252.

59. Kingdon C.C, Bowman E.W, Curran H, et al. Functional status and well-being in people with myalgic encephalomyelitis/chronic fatigue syndrome compared with people with multiple sclerosis and healthy controls. Pharmacoecon Open. 2018; 2: 381-392.

60. Nacul L C, Lacerda E M, Campion P, et al. The functional status and well being of people with myalgic encephalomyelitis/chronic fatigue syndrome and their carers. BMC Public Health. 2011; 11: 402

61. Núñez M, Núñez E, del Val J L, et al. Health-related quality of life in chronic fatigue syndrome versus rheumatoid arthritis as control group. J Chronic Fatigue Syndr. 2007; 14: 31-43

62. McIntyre, A, M.E.- Chronic Fatigue Syndrome: a practical guide. Thorsons, London 1998:1-33.

63. Halapy E, Parlor, M. The Quantitative Data: Environmental Sensitivities/Multiple Chemical Sensitivity (ES/MCS), Fibromyalgia (FM), Myalgic Encephalomyelitis/ Chronic Fatigue Syndrome (ME/CFS), October 2013. http://www.meao.ca/files/ Quantitative_Data_Report.pdf.

64. Ibid 3

Chapter 4 My Tipping Point

1. http://saME/CFS.asn.au/download/consensus_overview_me_ME/CFS.pdf (accessed March 2016)
2. Hoffman E, After Such Knowledge - a Meditation on the Aftermath of the Holocaust. Vintage London 2004.
3. Grinblat K (ed), Children of the Shadows: Voices of the Second-Generation. University of Western Australia Press, Crawley WA, 2002:61-6.

Chapter 5 ME/CFS Unmasked

1. https://www.mechanicalbasis.org/
2. Morris G, Maes M, Myalgic encephalomyelitis/chronic fatigue syndrome and encephalomyelitis disseminata/multiple sclerosis show remarkable levels of similarity in phenomenology and neuroimmune characteristics. BMC Med. 2013 Sep 17;11:205.
3. https://www.medicalnewstoday.com/articles/318586.php
4. Nakatomi Y, Mizuno K, Ishii A, Wada Y, Tanaka M, et al. Neuroinflammation in patients with will chronic fatigue syndrome/myalgic encephalomyelitis: an 11C-(R)-PK11195 PET study. J Nucl Med 2014;55:945–50.
5. Barnden LR, Crouch B, Kwiatek R, et al. Evidence in chronic fatigue syndrome for severity-dependent upregulation of prefrontal myelination that is independent of anxiety and depression. NMR Biomed. 2015 Mar;28(3):404-13.
6. Ibid 2
7. Ibid 5
8. Ibid
9. https://www.healthrising.org/blog/2020/07/11/mucosal-genes-chronic-fatigue-syndrome/
10. Craddock T, INIM ME/CFS Webinar May 15 2020. https://www.nova.edu/nim/events.html
11. Casado B, Pannell LK, Iadarola P, Baraniuk JN. Proteomics. 2005 Jul;5(11):2949-59.
12. Baraniuk JN, Petrie KN, Le U, Tai CF, et al. Neuropathology in rhinosinusitis. Am J Respir Crit Care Med. 2005 Jan 1;171(1):5-11.
13. Ibid 10
14. https://en.wikipedia.org/wiki/Gulf_War_syndrome
15. https://www.hopkinsmedicine.org/health/conditions-and-diseases/gulf-war-syndrome
16. Alshelh Z, Albrecht DS, Bergan C. et al In-vivo imaging of neuroinflammation in veterans with Gulf War illness. Brain Behav Immun. 2020 Feb 4. pii: S0889-1591(19)31334-0.

Chapter 6 Triggers

1. Perez M, Jaundoo R, Hilton K, et al. Genetic Predisposition for Immune System, Hormone, and Metabolic Dysfunction in Myalgic Encephalomyelitis/Chronic Fatigue Syndrome: A Pilot Study Front Pediatr. 2019 May 24;7:206.
2. Kaiser J, Biomedicine. Genes and chronic fatigue: how strong is the evidence? Science 2006;312(5774):669–71.
3. Buchwald D, Buchwald D, Hererell R, Ashton BS, Belcourt M, et al. A twin study of chronic fatigue. Psychosomatic Med 2001;63:936–43. 52.
4. Schur E, Afari N, Goldberg J, Dedra B, Sullivan PF. Twin analyses of fatigue. Twin Res Hum Genet 2007;10(5):729–33.

5. Hickie IB, Bansal AS, Kirk KM, Lloyd AR, Martin, NG. A twin study of the etiology of prolonged fatigue and immune activation. Twin Res 2001;4(2):94–102.
6. Bested AC, Marshall LM. Review of Myalgic Encephalomyelitis/Chronic Fatigue Syndrome: an evidence-based approach to diagnosis and management by clinicians. Rev Environ Health. 2015;30(4):231.
7. Dietert RR, Dietert JM. Possible role for early-life immune insult including developmental immunotoxicity in chronic fatigue syndrome (ME/CFS) or myalgic encephalomyelitis (ME). Toxicology. 2008 May 2;247(1):61-72.
8. Grinde B.Viruses belonging to Anelloviridae or Circoviridae as a possible cause of chronic fatigue J Transl Med. 2020; 18: 485.
9. Ibid
10. Lam M.H.-B.Mental morbidities and chronic fatigue in severe acute respiratory syndrome survivors: long-term follow-up. Arch Intern Med. 2009; 169: 2142-2147.
11. Moldofsky H. Patcai J. Chronic widespread musculoskeletal pain, fatigue, depression and disordered sleep in chronic post-SARS syndrome; a case-controlled study. BMC Neurol. 2011; 11: 37.
12. Mørch K, Hanevik K, Rivenes A.C., et al. Chronic fatigue syndrome 5 years after giardiasis: differential diagnoses, characteristics and natural course. BMC Gastroenterol. 2013; 13: 28.
13. De Venter M, Van Royen R, Moorkens G, et al. Differential effects of childhood trauma subtypes on fatigue and physical functioning in chronic fatigue syndrome. Comprehensive Psychiatry 2017;78: 76–82.
14. Yancey JR, Thomas SM, Chronic fatigue syndrome: diagnosis and treatment. Am Fam Physician. 2012 Oct 15;86(8):741-6.
15. Ibid 5
16. Mateo Cortes Rivera MC, Mastronardi C, Claudia T Silva-Aldana CT, et al. Myalgic Encephalomyelitis/Chronic Fatigue Syndrome: A Comprehensive Review. Diagnostics (Basel) 2019 Aug 7;9(3):91.
17. Hickie I, Davenport T, Wakefield D et al. Post-infective and Chronic Fatigue Syndromes Precipitated by Viral and Non-Viral Pathogens: Prospective Cohort Study BMJ. 2006 Sep 16;333(7568):575.
18. Ibid
19. ME/CFS The biomedical basis, diagnosis, treatment and management. International Research Symposium Geelong Australia, March 12-15.

Chapter 7 Long-COVID – the Growing Wave

1. Bateman L, Bested A C, Bonilla H F, et al. Myalgic Encephalomyelitis/Chronic Fatigue Syndrome: Essentials of Diagnosis and Management. Mayo Clinic Proceedings Consensus Recommendations. Open Access August 25, 2021. DOI:https//doi.org/10.1016/j.mayocp.2021.07.004 see full text link below:
    Read it here
2. Komaroff A.L, Bateman L. Will COVID-19 lead to myalgic encephalomyelitis/chronic fatigue syndrome? Front Med (Lausanne). 2021; 7: 606824
3. Ibid
4. US Centers for Disease Control and Prevention Post-COVID conditions. April 8, 2021:
5. https://www.cdc.gov/coronavirus/2019-ncov/long-term-effects.html
6. Kedor C, Freitag H, Meyer-Arndt L, et al. Chronic COVID-19 syndrome and chronic

fatigue syndrome (ME/CFS) following the first pandemic wave in Germany—a first analysis of a prospective observational study. medRxiv. Preprint posted online February 8, 2021.

7. https://doi.org/10.1101/2021.02.06.21249256
8. Ibid
9. Ibid 1
10. Ibid 1
11. Sommer SJ. ME/CFS - A Path Back to Life. Self published 2021 Available at www. drstevensommer.com.
12. Paul H. Covid-19 long-haulers and the experience of 'hidden' disabilities. Stat. October 7, 2020. https://www.statnews.com/2020/10/07/ covid-19-long-haulers-experience-hidden-disabilities/
13. Hickie I, Davenport T, Wakefield D et al. Post-infective and Chronic Fatigue Syndromes Precipitated by Viral and Non-Viral Pathogens: Prospective Cohort Study BMJ. 2006 Sep 16;333(7568):575.
14. Ibid 4
15. Ibid 5
16. Ibid 4
17. Ibid
18. https://www.bmj.com/content/371/bmj.m4938/rr
19. https://www.hopkinsmedicine.org/coronavirus/articles/icu-recovery.html
20. Ibid
21. https://www1.racgp.org.au/newsgp/clinical/ what-are-the-long-term-health-risks-post-covid-19.
22. Perrin R, Riste L, Hann M. Into the looking glass: Post-viral syndrome post COVID-19. Med Hypotheses. 2020 Nov; 144: 110055. Published online 2020 Jun 27. doi: 10.1016/j.mehy.2020.110055 PMCID: PMC7320866.\
23. Ngai JC, Ko FW, Ng SS, et al. The long-term impact of severe acute respiratory syndrome on pulmonary function, exercise capacity and health status. Respirology 2010; 15: 543–550. doi:10.1111/j.1440-1843.2010.01720.x
24. Tansey CM, Louie M, Loeb M, et al. One-year outcomes and health care utilization in survivors of severe acute respiratory syndrome. Arch Intern Med 2007; 167: 1312–1320. doi:10.1001/archinte.167.12.1312
25. Pavel A, Murray DK, Stoessl A J. COVID-19 and selective vulnerability to Parkinson's disease. The Lancet Neurology Correspondence| Volume 19, ISSUE 9, P719, September 01, 2020.
26. Whittaker A., Anson M., Harky A. Neurological Manifestations of COVID-19: A systematic review and current update. Acta Neurol. Scand. 2020;142(1):14–22. 25.Montalvan V. Neurological manifestations of COVID-19 and other coronavirus infections: a systematic review. Clin. Neurol. Neurosurg. 2020;194 p. 105921.
27. Neufeld KJ, Leoutsakos J-MS, Yan H, et al. Fatigue symptoms during the first year following ARDS. Chest 2020; in press [10.1016/j.chest.2020.03.059].
28. Kim H, Rebholz CM, Hegde S. Plant-based diets, pescatarian diets and COVID-19 severity: a population-based case–control study in six countries. BMJ Nutrition, June 07, 2021.
29. Ibid
30. Ibid 11
31. https://www.meaction.net/2020/07/10/dr-anthony-fauci-says-that-post-covid-syndrome-is-highly-suggestive-of-myalgic-encephalomyelitis/

32. https://www.marketwatch.com/story/by-far-the-worst-virus-i-have-ever-
     endured-olympic-gold-medalist-cameron-van-der-burgh-31-on-contracting-the-
     coronavirus-2020-03-24
33. Ibid 4
34. https://solveME/CFS.org/will-covid-19-leave-an-explosion-of-me-ME/
     CFS-cases-in-its-wake/
35. Consiglio C R, Cotugno N , Sardh F, et al The Immunology of Multisystem
     Inflammatory Syndrome in Children with COVID-19. Cell. 2020 Nov
     12;183(4):968-981.e7. doi: 10.1016/j.cell.2020.09.016. Epub 2020 Sep 6. Free PMC
     Article
36. 35.Li TS, Gomersall CD, Joynt GM, et al. Long-term outcome of acute respiratory
     distress syndrome caused by severe acute respiratory syndrome (SARS): an
     observational study. Crit Care Resusc. 2006 Dec;8(4):302-8.
37. Ibid
38. Lam MHB, Wing YK, Yu MWM, et al. Mental morbidities and chronic fatigue in
     severe acute respiratory syndrome survivors: long-term follow-up. Arch Int Med
     2009;169(22):2142-7.
39. Ibid
40. Moldofsky H, Patcaai J. Chronic widespread musculoskeletal pain, fatigue, depression
     and disordered sleep in chronic post-SARS syndrome; a case-controlled study BMC
     Neurol 2011. Mar 24;11 doi: 10.1186/1471-2377-11-37.
41. Ibid 35
42. Tan CW, Chia WN, Young BE, et al. Pan-Sarbecovirus Neutralizing Antibodies in
     BNT162b2-Immunized SARS-CoV-1 Survivors. August 18, 2021 DOI: 10.1056/
     NEJMoa2108453
43. Alwan N. A Negative COVID-19 Test Does not Mean Recovery. Nature Aug 13,
     2020;584:170.
44. Hickie I, Davenport T, Wakefield D et al. Post-infective and Chronic Fatigue
     Syndromes Precipitated by Viral and Non-Viral Pathogens: Prospective Cohort Study
     BMJ. 2006 Sep 16;333(7568):575.
45. 44.Sandler CX, Lloyd AR. Chronic fatigue syndrome: progress and possibilities Med J
     Aust 2020; 212 (9): . || doi: 10.5694/mja2.50553 Published online: 6 April 2020
46. Ibid 23
47. Ibid 24
48. Badrfam R. From encephalitis lethargica to COVID-19: Is there another epidemic
     ahead? Clin Neurol Neurosurg. 2020 Sep; 196: 106065.
49. https://www.svhs.org.au/research-education/participating-in-research-trials/
     adapt-study
50. Carfi A, Bernabei R, Gemelli F L. Persistent Symptoms in Patients After Acute
     COVID-19 [Against COVID-19 Post-Acute Care Study Group.] JAMA 2020 Aug
     11;324(6):603-605.
51. Zhao YM, Shang YM, Song WB, et al. Follow-up study of the pulmonary function
     and related physiological characteristics of COVID-19 survivors three months after
     recovery. EClinicalMedicine 25, 100463 (2020).
52. Wise J. Long covid: One in seven children may still have symptoms 15 weeks after
     infection, data show BMJ 2021 Sep 1;374:n2157. doi: 10.1136/bmj.n2157.
53. https://www.omf.ngo/
54. https://www.medpagetoday.com/special-reports/exclusives/91476

Chapter 8 My Experience/Cessation of Familiar Support (ME/CFS)

1. McIntyre, A, M.E.- Chronic Fatigue Syndrome: a practical guide. Foreword by Clare Francis. Thorsons, London 1998:ix-xii.
2. Green J, Romei J, Natelson BJ. Stigma and chronic fatigue syndrome. Journal of Chronic Fatigue Syndrome. 1999; 5:63–75.
3. Twemlow SW, Bradshaw SL Jr, Coyne L, Lerma BH. Patterns of utilization of medical care and perceptions of the relationship between doctor and patient with chronic illness including chronic fatigue syndrome. Psychological Reports. 1997; 80:643–659.
4. House JS, Landis KR, Umberson D. Social relationships and health. Science 1988;241(4865): –540–5.
5. Orth-Gomer K, Johnson J V, Social network interaction and mortality. A six-year follow-up study of a random sample of the Swedish population. Journal of Chronic Diseases 1987;40(10):949–57.
6. Berkman LA, Syme SL. Social networks, host resistance, and mortality: a nine year follow-up study of Alameda County residents. American Journal of Epidemiology 1979;109:186–204.
7. Ibid
8. Prins JB, Bos E, Huibers MJ, et al. Social support and the persistence of complaints in chronic fatigue syndrome. Psychother Psychosom. 2004;73(3):174-182.
9. Chalder T, Godfrey E, Ridsdale L, King M, Wessely S. Predictors of outcome in a fatigued population in primary care following a randomized controlled trial. Psychol Med. 2003;33(2):283-287.
10. Band R, Wearden A, Barrowclough C. Patient Outcomes in Association With Significant Other Responses to Chronic Fatigue Syndrome: A Systematic Review of the Literature. Clin Psychol (New York). 2015 Mar;22(1):29-46. Epub 2015 Mar 14.
11. http://www.cdc.gov/media/transcripts/t061103.htm [accessed March 2016]
12. https://nursingclio.org/2018/09/25/golden-girls-chronic-fatigue-syndrome-and-the-legacies-of-hysteria/ [Accessed March 2019]
13. Kingdon C.C,Bowman E.W, Curran H, et al. Functional status and well-being in people with myalgic encephalomyelitis/chronic fatigue syndrome compared with people with multiple sclerosis and healthy controls. Pharmacoecon Open. 2018; 2: 381-392.
14. Komaroff A L, Fagioli L R, Doolittle T.H, et al. Health status in patients with chronic fatigue syndrome and in general population and disease comparison groups. Am J Med. 1996; 101: 281-290.
15. Stein E. Chronic fatigue syndrome. Assessment and treatment of patients with ME/CFS: Clinical guidelines for psychiatrists. 2005.
16. https://s3.amazonaws.com/kajabi-storefronts-production/sites/90617/themes/1513565/downloads/TSGDbZnFSWOjdt3msZgv_Guidelines-Paper-English.pdf [Accessed: December 2020]
17. Hoffman E, After Such Knowledge - a Meditation on the Aftermath of the Holocaust. Vintage London 2004.
18. https://www.psycom.net/depression.central.grief.html
19. US Centers for Disease Control and Prevention Mental health and chronic diseases. CDC fact sheet. Issue Brief No. 2 October2012.https://www.cdc.gov/workplacehealthpromotion/tools-resources/pdfs/issue-brief-no-2-mentalhealth-and-chronic-disease.pdf [Accessed: December 2020]
20. http://www.ME/CFSselfhelp.org/library/26-grieving-your-losses [Accessed March 2020]

Chapter 9 A Carer's Reflection Tori Sommer

Chapter 10 Multisystem Malfunction - the Evidence
Pt 1 Mitochondrial Dysfunction and the Hibernation Switch

1.	https://www.bbc.co.uk/bitesize/guides/zm6rd2p/revision/
2.	http://www.vce.bioninja.com.au/aos-1-molecules-of-life/biochemical-processes/cell-respiration.html
3.	Morris G, Maes M. Mitochondrial dysfunctions in myalgic encephalomyelitis/chronic fatigue syndrome explained by activated immuno-inflammatory, oxidative and nitrosative stress pathways. Metab Brain Dis. 2014 Mar;29(1):19-36
4.	Keller B A, Pryor J L, Giloteaux L. Inability of myalgic encephalomyelitis/chronic fatigue syndrome patients to reproduce VO2peak indicates functional impairment.J Transl Med. 2014; 12: 104.
5.	Lien K, Johansen B, Marit B. Veierød, et al. Abnormal blood lactate accumulation during repeated exercise testing in myalgic encephalomyelitis/chronic fatigue syndrome. Physiology Reports Open Access 2019;7(11).
6.	Gerwyn M , Maes M. Mechanisms Explaining Muscle Fatigue and Muscle Pain in Patients with Myalgic Encephalomyelitis/Chronic Fatigue Syndrome (ME/CFS): a Review of Recent Findings 2017. Curr Rheumatol Rep. Jan;19(1):1.
7.	Tomas C, Newton J. Metabolic abnormalities in chronic fatigue syndrome/myalgic encephalomyelitis: a mini-review.Biochem Soc Trans. 2018; 46: 547-553.
8.	https://www.youtube.com/watch?v=kbaW4JKkin4
9.	https://www.youtube.com/watch?v=OFdKZ9jQtsA
10.	Naviaux RK, Naviaux JC, Li K, et al. Metabolic features of chronic fatigue syndrome. Proc Natl Acad Sci U S A. 2016 Sep 13;113(37):E5472-80.
11.	Ibid
12.	https://www.newscientist.com/article/2121162-metabolic-switch-may-bring-on-chronic-fatigue-syndrome/
13.	Hickie I, Davenport T, Wakefield D et al. Post-infective and Chronic Fatigue Syndromes Precipitated by Viral and Non-Viral Pathogens: Prospective Cohort Study BMJ. 2006 Sep 16;333(7568):575.
14.	O Fluge, Mella O, Bruland Ove, et al. Metabolic profiling indicates impaired pyruvate dehydrogenase function in myalgic encephalopathy/chronic fatigue syndrome. JCI Insight 2016 Dec 22;1(21):e89376.
15.	Ibid 11

Chapter 11 Multisystem Malfunction - the Evidence
Pt 2 Neuroendocrine and Autonomic Nervous System Dysfunction

1.	Mathew SJ, Mao X, Keegan KA, Levine SM, Smith ELP, et al. Ventricular cerebrospinal fluid lactate is increased in chronic fatigue syndrome compared with generalized anxiety disorder: an in vivo 3.0 T (1)H MRS imaging study. NMR Biomed 2009;22(3):251–8.
2.	Fuite J, Vernon SD, Broderick G. Neuroendocrine and immune network re-modeling in chronic fatigue syndrome: an exploratory analysis. Genomics 2008;92(6):393–9.
3.	Fletcher MA, Rosenthal M, Antoni M, Ironson G, Zeng XR, et al. Plasma neuropeptide Y: a biomarker for symptom severity in chronic syndrome. Behav Brain Funct 2010;6:76. 122. Papadopoulos AS, Cleare AJ. Hypothalamic-pituitary-

adrenal axis dysfunction in chronic fatigue syndrome. Nat Rev Endocrinol 2011 Sep;8(1):22–32.

4. De Becker P, De Meirleir K, Joos E, et al. Dehydroepiandrosterone (DHEA) response to i.v. ACTH in patients with chronic fatigue syndrome. Horm Metab Res 1999;31(1):18–21.

5. Allain TJ, Bearn JA, Coskeran P, et al. Changes in growth hormone, insulin, insulin like growth factors (IGFs), and IGF-binding protein-1 in chronic fatigue syndrome. Biol Psychiatry 1997 41(5):567–73.

6. Sharpe M, Clements A, Hawton K, et al. Increased prolactin response to Buspirone in chronic fatigue syndrome. J Affect Disord 1996;41(1):71–6.

7. Bakheit AM, Behan PO, Watson WS, et al. Abnormal arginine-vasopressin secretion and water metabolism in patients with postviral fatigue syndrome. Acta Neurol Scand 1993;87(3):234–8.

8. Boneva RS, Decker MJ, Maloney EM, et al. Higher heart rate and reduced heart rate variability persist during sleep in chronic fatigue syndrome: a population-based study. Auton Neurosci 2007;137(1–2):94–101.

9. Ibid

10. Davenport TE, Lehnen M, Stevens SR, et al. Chronotropic Intolerance: An Overlooked Determinant of Symptoms and Activity Limitation in Myalgic Encephalomyelitis/Chronic Fatigue Syndrome? Front Pediatr. 2019 Mar 22;7:82.

11. Lien K, Johansen B, Marit B, et al. Abnormal blood lactate accumulation during repeated exercise testing in myalgic encephalomyelitis/chronic fatigue syndrome. Physiology Reports Open Access 2019;7(11).

12. Ibid 10

Chapter 12 Multisystem Malfunction - the Evidence
Pt 3 Immune System Dysfunction

1. ME/CFS The biomedical basis, diagnosis, treatment and management. International Research Symposium Geelong Australia, March 12-15

2. Nijs J, Nees A, Paul L, et al., Altered immune response to exercise in patients with chronic fatigue syndrome/myalgic encephalomyelitis: a systematic literature review. Exerc Immunol Rev. 2014;20:94-116

3. White AT, Light AR, Hughen RW, Bateman L, Thomas B, et al. Severity of symptom flare after moderate exercise is linked to cytokine activity in chronic fatigue syndrome. Psychophysiology 2010;47(4):615–24.

4. https://nam.edu/

5. Siegel SD, Antoni MH, Fletcher MA, Maher K, Segota MC, et al. Impaired natural immunity, cognitive dysfunction, and physical symptoms in patients with chronic fatigue syndrome: Preliminary evidence for a subgroup? J Psychosom Res 2006;60(6):559–66.

6. Hornig M, MOntoya JG, Klimas NG, Levine S, Felsenstein D, et al. Distinct plasma immune signatures in ME/CFS are present early in the course of illness. Sci Adv 2015;1:e1400121.

7. Broderick G, Fuite J, Kreitz A, Vernonb SD, Klimas N, et al. A formal analysis of cytokine networks in chronic fatigue syndrome. Brain Behav Immun 2010;24(7):1209–17.

8. Fletcher MA, Zeng XR, Barnes Z, Leivs S, Klimas NG. Plasma cytokines in women with chronic fatigue syndrome. J Transl Med 2009;7:96.

9.   Fletcher MA, Zeng XR, Maher K, Levis S, Hurwitz B, et al. Biomarkers in chronic fatigue syndrome: Evaluation of natural killer cell function and dipeptidyl peptidase IV/CD26. PLoS ONE 2010;5(5):e10817.
10. Klimas NG, Salvato FR, Morgan R, Fletcher MA. Immunologic abnormalities in chronic fatigue syndrome. J Clin Microbiol 1990;28(6):1403–10.
11. Brenu EW, Huth TK, Hardcastle SL, Fuller K, Kaur M, et al. Role of adaptive and innate immune cells in chronic fatigue syndrome/ myalgic encephalomyelitis. Int Immun 2014;26(4):233–42.
12. Hardcastle SL, Brenu EW, Johnston S, Nguyen T, Huth T, et al. Characterization of cell functions and receptors in Chronic Fatigue Syndrome/Myalgic Encephalomyelitis (ME/CFS/ME). BMC Immunology 2015;16:35.
13. Stringer EA, Baker KS, Carroll IR, Montoya JG, Chu L, et al. Daily cytokine fluctuations, driven by leptin, are associated with fatigue severity in chronic fatigue syndrome: evidence of inflammatory pathology. J Translat Med 2013;11:93.
14. Potential Melastatin 3 Ion Channel Activity in Natural Killer Cells From Chronic Fatigue Syndrome/ Myalgic Encephalomyelitis Patients. Mol Med. 2019 Apr 23;25(1):14.
15. Ibid 6
16. Bested AC, Marshall LM. Review of Myalgic Encephalomyelitis/Chronic Fatigue Syndrome: an evidence-based approach to diagnosis and management by clinicians. Rev Environ Health. 2015;30(4):236.

Chapter 13 Beyond GET References

1.   https://vimeo.com/ondemand/klimasexercise
2.   https://nam.edu/
3.   Siegel SD, Antoni MH, Fletcher MA, Maher K, Segota MC, et al. Impaired natural immunity, cognitive dysfunction, and physical symptoms in patients with chronic fatigue syndrome: Preliminary evidence for a subgroup? J Psychosom Res 2006;60(6):559–66.
4.   Hornig M, MOntoya JG, Klimas NG, Levine S, Felsenstein D, et al. Distinct plasma immune signatures in ME/CFS are present early in the course of illness. Sci Adv 2015;1:e1400121.
5.   Stringer EA, Baker KS, Carroll IR, Montoya JG, Chu L, et al. Daily cytokine fluctuations, driven by leptin, are associated with fatigue severity in chronic fatigue syndrome: evidence of inflammatory pathology. J Translat Med 2013;11:93.
6.   White AT, Light AR, Hughen RW, Bateman L, Thomas B, et al. Severity of symptom flare after moderate exercise is linked to cytokine activity in chronic fatigue syndrome. Psychophysiology 2010;47(4):615–24.
7.   Nijs J, Nees A, Paul L, et al., Altered immune response to exercise in patients with chronic fatigue syndrome/myalgic encephalomyelitis: a systematic literature review. Exerc Immunol Rev. 2014;20:94-116
8.   https://www.theguardian.com/society/2020/nov/10/ fatigue-syndrome-exercise-therapy-loses-nice-recommendation
9.   Action for M.E. Severely neglected: M.E. in the U.K.—membership survey. London Action for M.E. Mar.2001 2:1–8. Available from: ttp://www.actionforme. org.uk/Resources/Action%20for %20ME/Documents/get-informed/Severely%20 Neglected%202001. (Accessed July 2019)
10. Kindlon T. Reporting of harms associated with graded exercise therapy and cognitive

behavioural therapy in myalgic encephalomyelitis/chronic fatigue syndrome. Bulletin of IACFS/ ME. 2011; 9(2):59–111.

11. Action for ME and Association of Young People with ME. ME 2008: What progress? May. 2008 Available at: http://www.actionforme.org.uk/Resources/Action%20 for %20ME/Documents/getinformed/ME%202008%20%20What%20progress. pdf(accessed July 2019)

12. Ibid 4.

13. Ibid 5

14. Ibid 6

15. Black CD, McCully KK. Time course of exercise induced alterations in daily activity in chronic fatigue syndrome. Dynamic Med 2005;4:10.10.1186/1476-5918-4-10.

16. Ibid

17. Wallman KE, Morton AR, Goodman C, Grove R, Guilfoyle AM. Randomized controlled trial of graded exercise in chronic fatigue syndrome. Medical Journal of Australia. 2004; 180:444–448.

18. Ibid

19. Larun L, Brurberg KG, Odgaard-Jensen J, Price JR. Exercise therapy for chronic fatigue syndrome. Cochrane Database Syst Rev. 2016 Feb 7;2:CD003200. doi: 10.1002/14651858.CD003200.pub4. Review.

20. Price JR, Mitchell E, Tidy E, Hunot V. Cognitive behaviour therapy for chronic fatigue syndrome in adults. Cochrane Database Syst Rev. 2008;(3):CD001027.

21. Ibid 8

22. Ibid 9

23. Ibid 10

24. White PD, Goldsmith KA, Johnson AL, et al.; PACE trial management group. Comparison of adaptive pacing therapy, cognitive behavior therapy, graded exercise therapy, and specialist medical care for chronic fatigue syndrome (PACE): a randomized trial. Lancet. 2011;377(9768):823-836.

25. Ibid

26. White P D, Goldsmith K, Johnson A L, et al. Recovery from chronic fatigue syndrome after treatments given in the PACE trial. Psychol Med. 2013; 43: 2227-2235.

27. Wilshire CE, Kindlon T, Courtney R et al. Rethinking the treatment of chronic fatigue syndrome-a reanalysis and evaluation of findings from a recent major trial of graded exercise and CBT. BMC Psychol 2018 Mar 22;6(1):6.

28. Marks D F."Special issue on the PACE trial" [erratum appears in J Health Psychol. 2018;23(1):139]. J Health psychol. 2017; 22: 1103-1105.

29. Ibid 26

30. https://me-pedia.org/images/8/89/PACE-get-therapist-manual.pdf

31. Ibid

32. Davenport TE, Lehnen M, Stevens SR, et al. Chronotropic Intolerance: An Overlooked Determinant of Symptoms and Activity Limitation in Myalgic Encephalomyelitis/Chronic Fatigue Syndrome? Front Pediatr. 2019 Mar 22;7:82.

33. Ibid 26

34. http://cfsrecoveryproject.com/ how-to-benefit-from-exercise-even-if-you-have-chronic-fatigue-syndrome/

35. Ibid 1.

36. https://www.healthrising.org/blog/2020/11/13/ nice discards graded-exercise-therapy-cbt-treatment-chronic-fatigue-syndrome/

Chapter 14 Epigenetic 'Switches'

1. https://www.shutterstock.com/search/dna+helix+with+A+T+C+G+black+and+white?kw=free+images&gclid=EAIaIQobChMIrO2_xbPb4gIVDhSPCh3XIwTcEAAYASAAEgKKNfD_BwE&gclsrc=aw.ds

2. Spector T. Identically different - Why you can change your genes. Weidenfeld & Nicholson 2012:9,10.

3. https://en.wikipedia.org/wiki/Genomics (accessed February 2019)

4. Ibid, 2, p11.

5. http://www.pbs.org/wgbh/nova/body/epigenetics.html (accessed February 2019)

6. http://learn.genetics.utah.edu/content/epigenetics/ (accessed February 2019)

7. Ibid, 2, p35.

8. Richardson K, The Making of intelligence. New York: Columbia University Press 2000. (Reference by Rossi EL, The Psychobiology of Gene Expression: Neuroscience and Neurogenesis in Hypnosis in the Healing Arts. New York: WW Norton and Co. 2002:50.)

9. Buchwald D, Buchwald D, Hererell R, Ashton BS, Belcourt M, et al. A twin study of chronic fatigue. Psychosomatic Med 2001;63:936–43.

10. Schur E, Afari N, Goldberg J, Dedra B, Sullivan PF. Twin analyses of fatigue. Twin Res Hum Genet 2007;10(5):729–33.

11. Hickie IB, Bansal AS, Kirk KM, Lloyd AR, Martin, NG. A twin study of the etiology of prolonged fatigue and immune activation. Twin Res 2001;4(2):94–102.

12. Kaiser J, Biomedicine. Genes and chronic fatigue: how strong is the evidence? Science 2006;312(5774):669–71.

13. Ibid. 2, p1-5.

14. MacGregor AJ, Snieder H, Rigby AS, et al. Characterizing the quantitative genetic contribution to rheumatoid arthritis using data from twins. Arthritis Rheum 2000 Jan;43(1):30-7.

15. Roos L, van Dongen J, Bell CG, et al. Integrative DNA methylome analysis of pan-cancer biomarkers in cancer discordant monozygotic twin-pairs. Clin Epigenetics. 2016 Jan 20;8:7. doi: 10.1186/s13148-016-0172-y. eCollection 2016.

16. Ibid. 2, p20

17. Jablonka E, Raz G. Transgenerational epigenetic inheritance: prevalence, mechanisms, and implications for the study of heredity and evolution. Q Rev Biol.2009 Jun;84(2):131-76. Review.

18. http://nutrigenomics.ucdavis.edu (accessed February 2016)

19. DeBusk R, Joffe Y. It's Not Just Your Genes! Your diet, your lifestyle, your genes. BKDR Inc. USA 2006:21-2.

20. DeBusk R, Genetics: The Nutrition Connection. Chicago IL: The American Dietetic Association, 2003.

21. Menendez JA, Vellon L, Colomer R, et al. Effect of gamma-linolenic acid on the transcriptional activity of the Her-2/neu (erbB- 2) oncogene. J Natl Cancer Inst 2005;97(21):1611-1615.

22. Dusek JA, Otu HH, Wohlhueter AL, et al. Genomic counter-stress changes induced by the relaxation response. PLoS One. 2008 Jul 2;3(7):e2576.

23. Ibid

24. Bhasin MK, Dusek JA, Chang BH et al. Relaxation response induces temporal transcriptome changes in energy metabolism, insulin secretion and inflammatory pathways. PLoS One. 2013 May 1;8(5):e62817.

25. Ornish D, Magbanua MJ, Weidner G, et al. Changes in prostate gene expression in men undergoing an intensive nutrition and lifestyle intervention. Proc Natl Acad Sci U S A. 2008 Jun 17;105(24):8369-74.

26. Ornish D, Lin J, Chan JM, et al. Effect of comprehensive lifestyle changes on telomerase activity and telomere length in men with biopsy-proven low-risk prostate cancer: 5-year follow-up of a descriptive pilot study, Lancet Oncol. 2013 Oct;14(11):1112-20.

27. Jellinek G. Taking Control of Multiple Sclerosis -- Natural and Medical Therapies to Prevent its Progression. Melbourne: Hyland House Publishing 2005.

28. Esparza ML, Sasaki S, Kesteloot H. Nutrition, latitude and Multiple Sclerosis mortality: an ecologic study. Am J Epidemiol 1995;142:733-7.

29. Swank RL, Dugan BB. Effect of low saturated fat diet in early and late cases of Multiple Sclerosis. Lancet 1990;336:37-9.

30. Swank RL. Multiple Sclerosis: fat-oil relationship. Nutrition 1991;7:368-76.

31. Hadgkiss EJ, Jelinek GA, Weiland TJ et al. Health-related quality of life outcomes at 1 and 5 years after a residential retreat promoting lifestyle modification for people with multiple sclerosis, Neurol Sci. 2013 Feb;34(2):187-95.

32. lifestylemedicine.com.au (accessed February 2019)

33. lifestylemedicine.org (accessed February 2019)

34. http://www.calmlifestylemedicine.ca/ (accessed September 2019)

35. eu-lifestyle medicine.org (accessed February 2019)

36. Egger GJ, Binns AF, Rossner SR. The emergence of 'lifestyle medicine' as a structured approach for management of chronic disease. Med J Aust 2009;190(3):143-145.

Chapter 15 Hope Knocks On Our Door

1. https://www.statnews.com/2017/09/25/chronic-fatigue-syndrome-cdc/

2. https://www.thelancet.com/journals/lancet/article/PIIS0140-6736(15)60270-7/fulltext

3. Nakatomi Y, Mizuno K, Ishii A, Wada Y, Tanaka M, et al. Neuroinflammation in patients with will chronic fatigue syndrome/myalgic encephalomyelitis: an 11C-(R)-PK11195 PET study. J Nucl Med 2014;55:945–50.

4. Davenport TE, Lehnen M, Stevens SR, et al. Chronotropic Intolerance: An Overlooked Determinant of Symptoms and Activity Limitation in Myalgic Encephalomyelitis/Chronic Fatigue Syndrome? Front Pediatr. 2019 Mar 22;7:82.

Epilogue

1. Bateman L, Darakjy S, Klimas N, et al. Chronic fatigue syndrome and co-morbid and consequent conditions: evidence from a multi-site clinical epidemiology study. Fatigue. 2015; 3: 1-15.

GLOSSARY OF ACRONYMS

ANTS	Automatic Negative Thoughts
CPET	Cardiopulmonary Testing
CI	Chronotropic Intolerance
CFS	Chronic Fatigue Syndrome
CFIDS	Chronic Fatigue Immune Deficiency Syndrome
NMH	Neurally Mediated Hypotension
ME	Myalgic Encephalomyelitis
MS	Multiple Sclerosis
NMH	Neurally Mediated Hypotension
OI	Orthostatic Intolerance
PD	Parkinson's Disease
PEM	Post-exertional malaise
PETS	Positive Emotional Thoughts
POTS	Postural Orthostatic Tachycardia Syndrome
RPE	Rating of Perceived Exertion (1 to10)
SARS	Severe Acute Respiratory Syndrome
SEID	Systemic Exertion Intolerance Disease

FURTHER RESOURCES

Websites Visit ME/CFS sites:

www.emerge.org.au (Accessed December 2020)
https://mecfs.org.au/ Australia (Accessed December 2020)
http://www.cfidsselfhelp.org/ USA (Accessed December 2020)
http://www.meassociation.org.uk/ UK (Accessed December 2020)

Other Links

www.drstevensommer.com
https://lewisinstitute.com.au/ (Accessed December 2020)
https://www.healthrising.org/ (Accessed December 2020)
https://phoenixrising.me/ (Accessed December 2020)
https://www.betterhealth.vic.gov.au/health/conditionsandtreatments/
chronic-fatigue-syndrome-cfs (Accessed December 2020)
https://www.sbs.com.au/ondemand/video/1334946883764/insight-
chronic-fatigue-syndrome (Accessed December 2020)

Fact Sheets

https://emerge.org.au/category/about-mecfs/fact-sheets/#.
Xdo4BtVS8dc
Includes fact sheets on diagnosis, management, pacing, research and
explanations for family and friends.

Books

Barton A. Recovery from CFS – 50 personal stories. Author House UK
Ltd 2008.

McIntyre A. Chronic Fatigue Syndrome – a practical guide. Thorsons
London 1998:1-33.

Vallings R. The Pocket Guide to Chronic Fatigue Syndrome ME – Key Facts and Tips for Improved Health. Calico Publishing 2017, Auckland.

Vallings R. Chronic Fatigue Syndrome ME - Symptom, Diagnosis, Management. Calico Publishing 2012, Auckland.

Campbell B. The Patient's Guide to Chronic Fatigue Syndrome and Fibromyalgia. 2011 Available at: http://www.cfidsselfhelp.org/library/the-patients-guide-chronic-fatigue-syndromefibromyalgia

Lynch A, Blucher P. Taking Nothing For Granted. A sportsman's fight against Chronic Fatigue. Harper Collins 2005. eBook available from Harper.

Sommer SJ. Finding Hope - when facing serious disease. Inspiring Stories, Healing Insights and Health Research. Amazon.com 2017. Also available from www.drstevensommer.com

Marchant J. Cure. Text publishing Melbourne 2016.

Look up ME/CFS Clinics in your local area or nearest city like:

https://lewisinstitute.com.au/ (Accessed December 2020)
https://activehealthclinic.com.au/about-us/ (Accessed December 2020)
http://www.austin.org.au/Adult_CFS (Accessed December 2020)
https://www.epworth.org.au/Our-Services/rehabilitation/Pages/chronic-fatigue-program.aspx (Accessed August 2020)
https://www.alfredhealth.org.au/services/chronic-fatigue-clinic (Accessed August 2020)
https://www.statnews.com/2017/09/25/chronic-fatigue-syndrome-cdc/
https://www.medpagetoday.com/rheumatology/generalrheumatology/78944

www.ingramcontent.com/pod-product-compliance
Lightning Source LLC
Chambersburg PA
CBHW030243030426
42336CB00009B/231